D0241929

a year with
james wong

GROW YOUR OWN
DRUGS

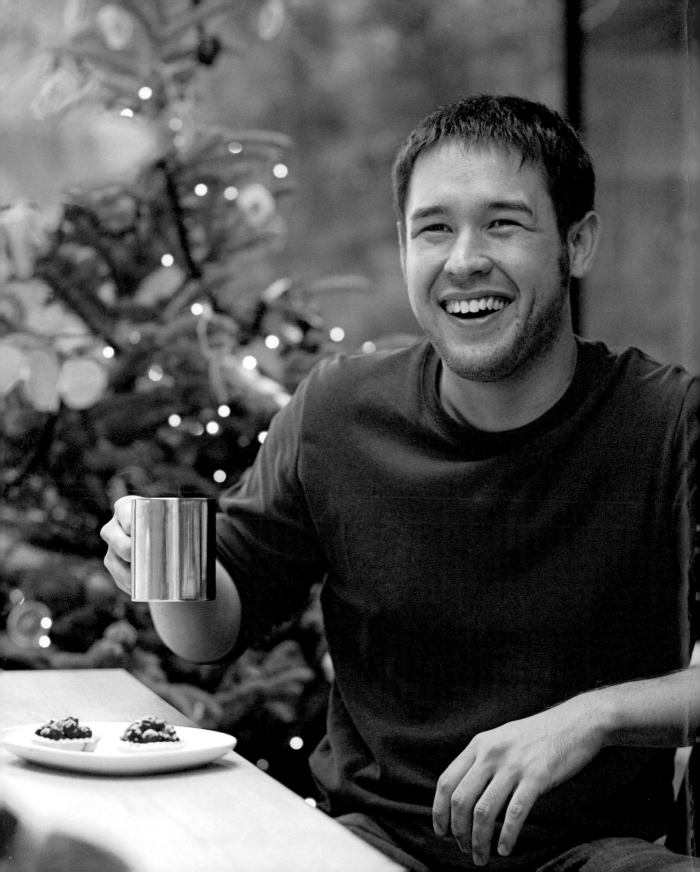

a year with james wong

GROW YOUR OWN
DRUGS

Collins

First published in 2010 by
Collins, an imprint of
HarperCollins*Publishers*
77-85 Fulham Palace Road
Hammersmith
London W6 8JB

www.collins.co.uk
www.harperplus.com/jameswong

Collins is a registered trademark of HarperCollins*Publishers* Ltd

10 9 8 7 6 5 4 3 2 1

Text © Silver River Productions Limited 2010
Commissioned photography © Cristian Barnett 2010

All rights reserved. No part of this publication may be reproduced,
stored in a retrieval system or transmitted, in any form or by
any means, electronic, mechanical, photocopying, recording
or otherwise, without the prior permission of the publishers.

A catalogue record for this book is available from the British Library.

ISBN 978 0 00 734530 4

Printed and bound by Butler Tanner & Dennis in Somerset, UK

Text Jane Phillimore
Commissioned Photography Cristian Barnett
Design and Art Direction Steve Boggs
Cover Design Nick Shah
Editor Caroline Curtis
Food Stylists Annie Rigg, Catherine Hill and Joy Skipper
Stylists Jo Harris, Lizzie Chambers
Consultant Liz Williamson, Professor of Pharmacy,
University of Reading
Horticultural Adviser Louise Danks, with thanks to Michael Kerr
Additional recipes Richard Adams, Hananja Brice Ytsma,
Nathalie Chidley, Lynne Hulka, Marcos Patchett, Neil Pellegrini
and Lorraine Wood, all of the Archway Clinic of Herbal Medicine
(www.archwayherbal.co.uk). Practitioners at the Archway Clinic
of Herbal Medicine are registered with the National Institute of
Herbal Medicine (NIHM).
Recipe Tester Nathalie Chidley

This edition of *Grow Your Own Drugs: A Year With James Wong* is interactive. Throughout the book you'll find symbols – these indicate that there are free extras available to you online.

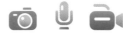

Simply visit www.harperplus.com/jameswong and enter the relevant page number. You can then access lots of extra content: see James talking about his remedies in videos and listen to his audio commentary, plus view great additional images.

DISCLAIMER

Please be aware that the advice given in this book is not intended as a replacement for professional medical treatment and advice. Do not diagnose or medicate yourself or others without first seeking medical advice. We strongly advise you to consult a medical practitioner before using any of these remedies, especially if you have an existing medical condition, are taking medication, are pregnant or are breastfeeding.

Do not use any remedies on children under the age of two, and check the cautions on specific remedies before using on older children.

Some herbs may interact with prescription drugs, including but not limited to the Pill and anti-depressants; you should always consult with a qualified medical practitioner before taking these remedies.

For remedies you put on the skin, always do a 24-hour skin test before using to check for allergies. There are some recipes with specific recommendations, so please be sure to follow those.

The case histories are not taken from clinical trials and cannot be considered proof of a remedy's efficacy, as results can be influenced by many factors.

The publishers and author do not accept responsibility for any loss, harm or damage that may result from your use or misuse of this book or your failure to seek appropriate medical advice.

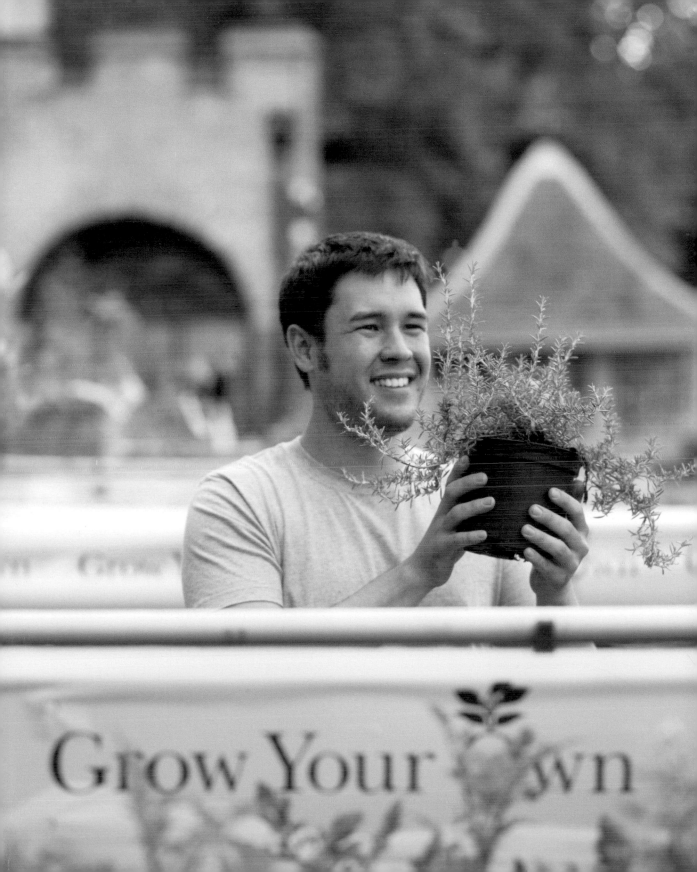
Grow Your own

CONTENTS

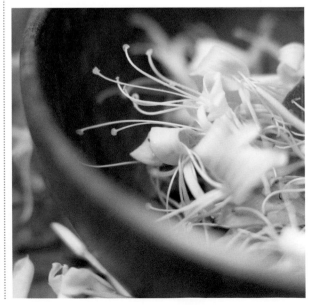

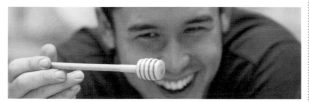
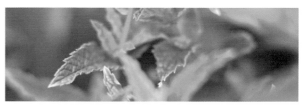
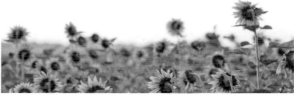
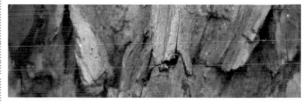
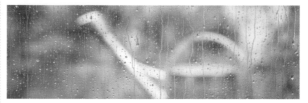

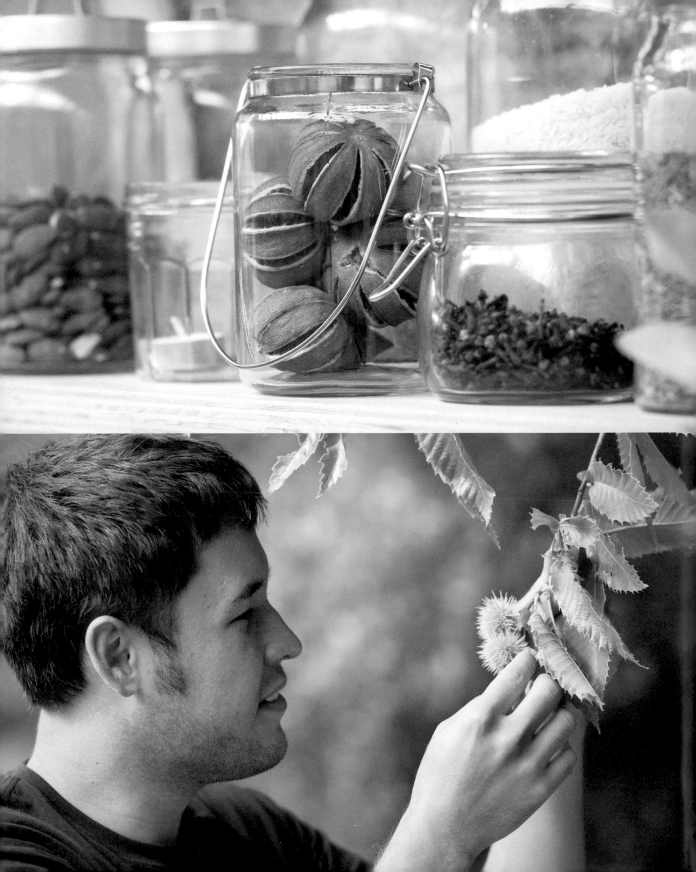

THE LIFE OF AN ETHNOBOTANIST!

1 THE LIFE OF AN ETHNOBOTANIST!

'Ethnobotanist' might not be the catchiest of job titles, and is guaranteed to incite confused looks on immigration forms, but though it sounds techy it describes what is – in my admittedly biased opinion – the most exciting, rewarding job in the world.

Once you start thinking about plants as solutions to problems in life, not just as a colourful backdrop to it, then even the dullest supermarket car park, council roundabout or urban front garden is transformed into a repository of fascinating chemicals, with direct genetic links to peoples and far-flung lands all over the world. And the best thing about it is that everyone can take part, simply by sprinkling a couple of seeds in a pot, raiding the local hedgerows or even foraging the shelves of the local supermarket.

Whether we know it or not, we rely on plants to provide almost everything around us: the food we eat, the clothes we wear, the medicines we take and – without sounding too eco about it – the very air we breathe. A leaflet from the Eden Project has a wonderful way of putting this: every material thing that is not mined, it says, is grown, a point that makes the relevance of plants to everyday life suddenly very clear. How exciting, how adventurous it is to discover for the first time the great impact plants have on us all. With so many of the big questions in life now answered, the wildernesses mapped and the mysteries solved, the amazing, undiscovered uses of plants seem to me to be one of the last great fields of exploration. Even after centuries of study, we still don't know exactly how many plant species exist, and with the best estimates hovering at over 300,000, there is no end to the potential for them to shock, surprise and delight us.

There is a tendency to think that the use of plants for medical purposes is something from history, making for an interesting anecdote rather than cutting-edge science. The reality could not be further from the truth. The world's largest and most lucrative pharmaceuticals market is the United States, where 70% of new medicinal drugs have been developed from natural sources. It is clear that we as a species are as reliant on the world of plants as we have ever been: plants are being used to create space-age plastics, ozone-saving biofuels, living pumps for drawing toxins out of soils contaminated by industry, and even giant underwater islands of seaweed to protect tropical coasts from tsunamis. Far from being over, our relationship with plants has only just begun.

And here's the great news: to take part in the revolution, all you need is a bit of earth, a pack of seeds and a tiny bit of know-how. You don't even need a garden: the concoctions won't mind where you source your ingredients. The backyards of friends and neighbours are my favourite source for botanical raw material; you'll be surprised how generous people will be when promised a jar of sticky sweet winter tonic or fragrant body scrubs in return for a few leaves and twigs. Newbies need not worry too much, either: simply follow a few hard and fast rules and make sure you know what you are picking and how to use it.

In this book, I hope to provide you with a complete tool kit that will get you off to a great start. Before you know it, you'll be tinkering away like a botanical Willy Wonka, mixing, matching and creating all manner of homespun goodies from the plants growing all around you.

And to help make it as easy as possible, I've got more tips, advice and variations relating to my remedies online at www.harperplus.com/jameswong. When you see the icons below, simply enter the page number on the website and you'll be taken directly to the material that complements the remedy you're reading about. The different icons indicate whether it is related video, audio or images.

Good luck – and have fun!

James Wong

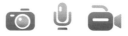 www.harperplus.com/jameswong

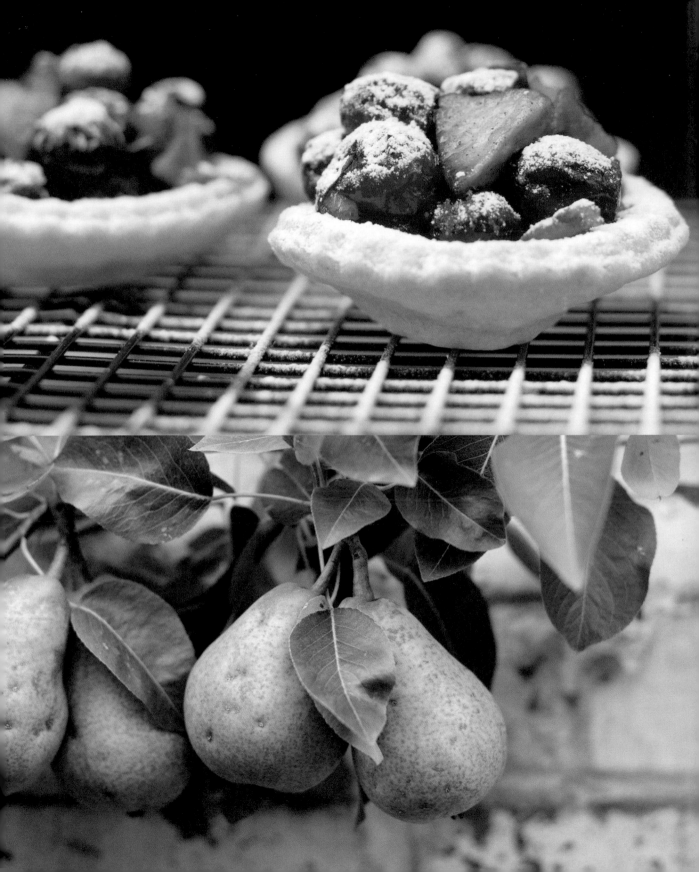

2 THE BASICS: GROWING AND MAKING

2 THE BASICS: GROWING AND MAKING

If some glossy cosmetics ads with their slick marketing spiel are to be believed, the makers of natural remedies must trek up the Amazon to find the rarest botanical ingredients, then prepare them in state-of-the-art laboratories belonging to huge Swiss institutes. So it is entirely understandable why so many people are daunted just by the idea of making home remedies. Fortunately, the romantic stories of marketing men, though they might make for beautiful TV adverts and entertaining reading, are very far from the truth.

More than three-quarters of the world relies on plants as the primary form of healthcare, and plant-based remedies have evolved as cheap, simple and easy-to-prepare solutions for people with very little time, resources or money. It is for this reason that I passionately believe plant-based remedies to be as relevant for our society as they are for shamans in the Andes or farmers in Malaysia. The average kitchen in the United Kingdom is infinitely better equipped than my gran's back in Borneo, where she would effortlessly whip up all manner of lotions and potions in mere minutes, from what were effectively the hedge trimmings out of the back garden. With mod cons like blenders, microwaves and dishwashers at our disposal, it is much quicker and easier for us to rustle up a recipe – no matter how domestically challenged we think we are. In this section I reveal a few tricks of the trade, which I hope will help demystify the growing side of things, and a couple of simple rules to ensure flawless concoctions every time.

It never fails to surprise me how many people seem utterly convinced they have some kind of superhero-like ability to kill plants. Please don't worry: pruning techniques needn't be perfect, and cultivation doesn't need to be absolutely spot on to get a plant to thrive well. In fact, to my mind the single most important rule in gardening, and one which is hardly ever mentioned, is that it is in a plant's own interest to grow. Plants have been around for millions of years without any help from humans and have independently evolved a huge range of ingenious strategies to cope with even the harshest conditions. As long as you place them in an environment that roughly matches the conditions they originally come from, they honestly are quite happy to take care of themselves – with little or no intervention from green (or not so green) fingers. In this section, I outline exactly how to identify your garden type – trust me, this is much more straightforward than it sounds! – and which plants are most likely to succeed in the conditions you have. If you get these two bits right, that's half the battle won.

As for herb plants, it's a wonderful coincidence that these happen to be the easiest of all plants to grow. Having originally evolved as weedy species that spring up on any piece of disturbed ground, they are perfectly happy to put up with all kinds of punishment, with many thriving on pure neglect.

If you've ever planted mint, lemon balm or feverfew, for example, you'll know that as soon as they're in the ground they spread rampantly, colonizing any bare earth and even cracks in the pavement. They won't need anything more than the occasional hacking back, giving you limitless handfuls for flavouring foods, concocting remedies and crafting cosmetics.

To transform your backyard clippings into a whole range of natural remedies, I also hope to demystify words like 'tincture', 'decoction' and 'salve', showing you how these can all be knocked up with only a few minutes' effort, with results rivalling anything to be found on the shelves of even the most upmarket health food shops and cosmetics counters.

GROWING
GROWING YOUR OWN PHARMACY

If you've never made a recipe in your life before, this book is a great place to start. And if you've never grown a plant before, even better. I want to cast away the dusty stereotypes that too often surround gardening, and in particular herbal remedies, and show you just how easy it is to get out there and start cultivating your very own living pharmacy – even if you are convinced you are a non-gardener. With just a couple of clippings from your backyard, you can create simple remedies for everyday ailments, spa-like beauty treatments and other practical products that bring a shine to furniture, scent to your home, or even get rid of your cat's fleas.

Nowadays, getting hold of medicinal plants and seeds is becoming ever easier. Even the most run-of-the-mill garden centres now stock a surprisingly broad range of the plants you need for just a couple of pounds. More than just the traditional parsley, sage and thyme, too: even my local high-street florist sells such weird and wonderful things as blackcurrant-scented sage, pineapple mint and Japanese wasabi plants (the source of the spicy green paste that accompanies sushi). Of course, once you have many of these planted up in your garden or window box, they often spread themselves all over the place via underground runners or seeds, popping up in even the most unexpected of places. But the most exciting thing about medicinal plants is that so many of these are common culinary ingredients: you need only look at the back of your refrigerator or spice rack for the plants you need. Simply pop a leftover stick of lemongrass in a glass of water on a window sill, or sprinkle a couple of grains from that jar of fennel seeds in a pot of compost, and in just a couple of months you will have a supply of fresh, organic, air mile-free ingredients for all sorts of remedies.

The tricky thing about so much choice, however, is that it can seem enormously daunting for a beginner. Where on earth do you start? The best way to simplify the whole business is just to pick plants that are useful at treating the afflictions you are prone to (see page 25) and which have a scent or flavour you like. As there is almost always a selection of several different plants that share similar properties, you have the luxury of picking and choosing whichever one(s) you like the most for a particular ailment.

Now, if you have never tried angelica, tansy or lemon balm before, let alone know what they look like, I have a simple recommendation: look round your local public botanic or herb garden; you'll find it's a great source of 'scratch and sniff' inspiration. Walking beside the beds and borders, you can get to know the look, smell and habit of plants you may otherwise have only read about in books or seen on TV, with neat little labels to guide you along the way, to decide which you like best. My favourite such garden is the Chelsea Physic Garden, just down the road from me, amidst the hustle and bustle of central London. It's hidden behind high walls, and you'll think you've stumbled across a small piece of undiscovered land, though it's actually been a virtual theme park for medicinal plant enthusiasts for more than three centuries; it was set up in 1673 to teach the doctors of the Royal Hospital, at a time when botany was a necessary part of medical training. Here, little labels dot the borders and, in true Harry Potter style, explain the plants' uses — 'once used by the Aztecs for dye', for example, and 'used to treat malaria'.

By keeping your eyes out at local gardens like these, you can pick up invaluable tips on what will grow well in your own backyard. If you spot a creeper thriving on a south-facing wall, for example, it is likely to do the same in a similar site at home for you. Conversely if you see a bush looking a bit forlorn in a boggy patch, you might want to think twice about planting it around your pond at home. This way, you are learning from the experiences of others; think of it as horticultural espionage.

I am passionate that plant-based medicine is so much more than its stereotype – a bit namby pamby, a bit hippy-ish. It deserves more respect than that: many contain powerful chemical ingredients and should therefore be treated with as much respect as conventional drugs. Plants can genuinely be a useful way to treat all sorts of minor, everyday complaints, but it is vital that you first receive a professional medical diagnosis, especially if you have an underlying medical condition, are taking medication, or are pregnant. If you think you may be sensitive to any of the ingredients, do a 24-hour skin test first to check for allergies. It is also important to use common sense when using plant-based remedies: don't give any of the remedies to children under the age of 2, or to children under 16 unless specified as safe in the recipe. (See also the special section for 'Kids', page 145).

But enough of that. Let's get started. Your own living pharmacy is just a few steps away.

GROWING:
IDENTIFY YOUR GARDEN TYPE

I've never been a slave to strict horticultural rules & regulations. That said, the textbooks do have some good advice; the most important point to note is that you should spend a little time in getting to know your site. To put it simply, if you understand the growing conditions of your site and pick your plants accordingly, gardening can be transformed. A never-ending labour and struggle against nature becomes a simple matter of a splash of water now and again as you pop out to forage in the flower border. In this section, I outline how to determine the specific conditions of your own site, be it rolling estate or window box, and show you how to work with, not against, your local conditions to get the best possible results.

Your garden's microclimate

Probably the single most important factor that influences what will grow best in your site is its climate. Each plot – no matter how small – has its own unique microclimate.

We may all complain about the British weather – and let's be fair, it isn't exactly southern California – but the United Kingdom nevertheless has the mildest climate of any place at an equivalent latitude either side of the Equator. This enables us to grow an enormous range of plants, which gardeners in many other parts of the world can only dream about. Why? Well, here comes the science: this unusual climate is produced because our weather is heavily influenced by the warm Gulf Stream current that flows up from the tropical Atlantic, bathing our island in a blanket of mild, wet air. This protects us from the harsh winters experienced by continental cities such as Moscow, but also gives us soggy, mild summers for which we are world-renowned. The further west you go in the country, the stronger the influence of this system, which is why most of Cornwall, south-west Ireland and western Scotland are so well suited to growing subtropical species like sun-loving acacias and lush tree ferns. Interestingly, the natural ecosystem of much of these regions was once temperate rainforest, much like that covering New Zealand, Chile, south-west China and the western coast of North America. Picking plants native to the mist-shrouded forests of these regions makes an excellent bet if you live out west.

On the flip side of things, the further east you go, the more the climate is influenced by the continent. Without the mediating force of the Atlantic, there are much wider extremes of temperature. Summers here are sunnier and drier, but winters are colder – with the possible exception of London, which has a unique climate all of its own. Like most big cities, London's urban sprawl traps heat and releases it slowly at night, which means it rarely – if ever – suffers major frosts, the centre being several degrees warmer than the surrounding countryside. With its comparatively low rainfall and greater amount of sunlight, the east and particularly the south-east is a good place to grow drought-tolerant, Mediterranean-type species since it has a broadly similar climate (more or less; I'm allowing myself a little artistic licence). Interestingly, the north–south divide is far less pronounced in our small island; there are warmer summers the further south you go, but that's about it.

In this section, I describe four specific types of microclimate that are typical of gardens in the United Kingdom, and suggest the kinds of plants that are suited to each. These are, of course, just examples; you may have a site that is exactly the same as one of the types described here, but the chances are that it is a combination of two or more. As in those magazine personality tests, there are no hard-and-fast rules, but identifying roughly the type of plot you have will make gardening a whole lot easier.

Type I – City-centre gardens and the far south-west
It might sound strange to lump the gardens of urban Hackney estates and quaint Cornish cottages together in the same category, but there is method to my madness: city-centre spaces and the far south-west enjoy similar growing conditions – some of the best in the whole country, in fact.

City-centre gardens are often considerably warmer than those of the surrounding countryside, the concrete jungle acting as a giant heat trap to shake off frost. The larger the city, the warmer its centre, which means that all over central London subtropical trees like avocados and citrus are a plausible option for die-hard exotic fans like me. The same concrete 'hot-water bottle' phenomenon applies to the domestic garden too: the closer a plant is positioned to a large wall (particularly a sunny south-facing one), the greater the protection it has from the cold. This is a trick that has been used since Victorian times to improve the growth of semi-tropical plants and even boost fruit and flower production on entirely hardy trees. The only key difficulties here are the size of plot needed – growing a

30m eucalyptus tree may not be very practical – and the potentially hazardous effect caused by very high pollution. A fact not often mentioned is that plants can absorb the toxic heavy metals from exhaust fumes, which are then concentrated in their tissues. Because of the potential effects of these, avoid eating plants that have been grown in extremely heavily polluted areas (close to a six-lane motorway, for example). Common sense is always the best rule of thumb; most urban dwellers are fine to get growing and eating.

In the far west and south-west of the country, similar conditions are achieved without the need for urban sprawl, and the extra rainfall and air humidity combine to create almost greenhouse-perfect growing conditions. This means that gardens abandoned for decades – such as the recently restored Trebah Gardens and Lost Gardens of Heligan – thrived for close to a century with almost no intervention from gardeners, though they were buried beneath a thorny forest of brambles. If there were only a Chinatown nearby, I'd be moving straight away!

In these conditions, you can grow the widest range of plants in the country, so you can pretty much take your pick. Gardeners on these sites are at a great advantage for growing tender species that would be impossible to grow anywhere else, and they also have the ideal conditions for growing most species native to the United Kingdom. The small handful of species that are at a slight disadvantage here are species that require frost to produce a good crop, such as blackcurrants and gooseberries. Luckily, these are few and far between.

Type 2 – Blustery hilltop spaces

Apart from the chance of having an amazing view from your deck chair, a hilltop garden can be a mixed blessing. Situated above the shelter of trees, buildings or indeed other hills, these gardens can suffer from strong winds, which can damage plants, either directly or by drying out the soil. The latter can exacerbate the tendency for hilltop gardens to be rather dry anyway, as rainfall drains quickly off these high places. In these conditions, delicate-leaved or moisture-loving plants (such as weeping willows) are unlikely to fare well. On the other hand, drought-tolerant, hard-leaved species (such as rosemary, lavender and thyme) will really shine. The good news for hilltop gardeners is that many of the most common medicinal plants come from Mediterranean climates, which means they thrive on dry soil and will cope well in windy conditions.

In situations such as these, protection from winds can radically improve growing conditions, and can be as simple as putting up a slatted fence or even just planting a simple evergreen hedge. Either solution will lessen the impact of wind damage and, in doing so, allow a much broader range of plants to be grown.

Digging a bit of organic matter (such as compost, leaf litter, even leftover vegetable peelings which have been rotted down in a compost bin) into the soil can greatly improve its ability to retain water on dry hilltop sites, the organic fibre acting exactly like a sponge.

It is not all bad news, however. Counterintuitive though this may seem, hilltop sites often enjoy far less cold and fewer frosts than surrounding gardens. The reason is simple: cold air sinks, meaning that wintery air drains freely off gardens on elevated sites and whisks away the chances of frost as it goes. If the garden is in the south of England, or even just faces south, this effect is even greater. Of course, if the hill we are talking about is of Alpine proportions these benefits start to diminish, but for most hills under about 400m above sea level (which is pretty high by UK standards) there is a definite benefit.

Type 3 – Lowland frost pockets

As mentioned above, dense cold air has a habit of running downhill, and if you live at the bottom of a hill, the accumulation of this chilly air can create intensely frosty conditions. This is particularly true in valleys and ditches, where frosts often arrive earlier and end later, making winters not only colder but also in effect making them last longer. This means that many of the more tender plants can find it difficult to survive in these areas. Rest assured that British native species – perfectly adapted to freezing cold winters – will grow away as if nothing ever happened.

Every cloud has a silver lining, however. Lowland frost pockets are often sheltered from the full effects of strong drying winds and are also less likely to suffer in times of drought   water, like cold air, flows downhill. This makes them a great place to grow hardy, moisture-loving species like marshmallow, willow, cranberries, angelica, meadowsweet, watermint and comfrey (great for making organic fertilizer).

Type 4 – Seafront sites

As the palm trees (*Phoenix canariensis, Trachycarpus fortunei, Chamaerops humilis*) that increasingly line seaside resort promenades attest, coastal gardens enjoy mild, sometimes even frost-free winters. Generally, the closer they are to the sea, the lower the chance of frost. They also have the rather dubious honour of being amongst the wettest places in the United Kingdom (with the exception of coastal Norfolk, Suffolk, Essex and Kent), but from a gardener's perspective this does mean very little watering is ever necessary. They also tend to be relatively well drained because most coastal sites have a sandy, friable soil, which means this extra rainfall does not result in the waterlogged soil that so many medicinal plants, and particularly herbs, hate.

These wonderfully mild conditions do come at a price, however, in the form of the huge gusts of salt-laden winds that blow in off the sea, especially in the winter months. Such winds can have a particularly damaging effect on plants, particularly soft, leafy species. Despite this, and with a few cleverly planted trees or hedges to act as windbreaks, you can create a space that enjoys the best of both worlds: mild, moist conditions sheltered from the full force of the winds. Abbotsbury Subtropical Gardens on the south coast is a perfect example, where a dense barrier of evergreen trees have created a sheltered microclimate with stunning results.

Soil science

Apart from planting wind breaks or creating heat-retaining walls, there is not an awful lot you can do to significantly change the climate of your site (short of building an enormous Eden Project-style dome over it). You can, however, radically improve your growing conditions – by improving your soil.

Soil quality has a direct impact on the health of your plants. By making small adjustments to this, you can dramatically change not only how well your plants grow but even which species it is possible to grow on your site.

To improve it, you first need to figure out what kind of soil you have, and the good news is you don't need a 'CSI'-style lab to analyse it. Just grab a handful of soil on a dry day and give it a good squeeze. Then ask yourself:

A Does the soil break up easily, feel a bit gritty, and filter through your fingers?
B Does the soil clump together, look slightly shiny, and roll easily into a firm sausage shape?
C Does the soil roll into a loose, fragile, sausage shape?

A It's sandy soil

Many Mediterranean-type herbs and plants (fennel, lavender, lemon verbena, olive, rosemary, scented-leaved pelargoniums, thyme) thrive on this kind of soil because it is as close as possible to that of their native environment, to which they are perfectly adapted. Being wonderfully free-draining, this type of soil does not suffer from waterlogging and is extremely well aerated.

While many plants love this soil, there is a major down side to its open, friable texture: water and nutrients tend to drain straight through it. This means that it can often hold too little of these essential elements to support the healthy growth of many species that aren't specifically adapted to cope in these harsh conditions.

There is, however, a very simple way to greatly improve the water- and nutrient-holding capacity of sandy soil: every year, apply a good layer of organic matter (compost, leaf litter, well-rotted manure or even just leftover vegetable peelings which have been rotted down in a compost bin). This organic matter acts like a sponge to retain water and the nutrients dissolved in it, and make it available to the roots of plants. If you want to, feel free to dig the matter in, but this is not strictly necessary. (If you're wondering why, see 'To dig or not to dig' below for a full explanation.)

B It's clay soil

When the tiny particles of clay meet water, they stick together, making this soil clumpy and heavy. This makes it far superior to sandy soil in terms of its excellent water- and nutrient-retaining properties, but its dense, pastelike consistency can restrict the flow of air to, and the uptake of nutrients by, the plant's roots. Many half-hardy plants that do not survive the winter are not necessarily the victims of the cold itself but instead succumb to the stifling effects of waterlogged soil, which cause bacterial or fungal infections that rot the roots. Clay soils also have a tendency to bake rock hard in hot, dry summers, just like pottery in a kiln, leaving your plants struggling to grow in what is almost a natural concrete.

Just like sandy soil, the addition of organic matter every year will greatly improve the condition of heavy clay soil. Here the fibrous texture of organic materials like compost or leaf litter opens up the soil structure and allows air in. Additionally, digging in some grit or horticultural sand will break up the heavy clods to improve drainage. (Whatever you do, though, please don't use builder's or beach sand, which contain plant-damaging lime or salt.) You'll find that the soil becomes freer-flowing and less likely to waterlog, with a texture more like the topping of an apple crumble than dense cookie dough, which gives plants a far better chance.

C It's loamy soil

Congratulations! You have the soil type that all other gardeners want, the perfect mixture of water- and nutrient-retaining clay and friable, well-drained sand. You get different variations of this (more clay than sand, more sand than clay), but on the whole this soil is ideal for growing the widest range of plants. Having said this, excellence can always be improved upon, and (again) this is achieved by piling on the organic matter every year to keep the nutrient levels high.

To dig or not to dig?

The first point to note is that garden compost, leaf mould, well-rotted manure or other bulky fertilizers are all considered to be organic matter; granules, pellets or liquid feeds aren't.

Now, adding organic matter to soil aerates and enriches it, but there is a big debate about whether you should dig it in, or just leave it on the surface and let the worms do the work for you. Being a resolutely lazy gardener, I prefer the second option. Shovel on a load of organic matter in autumn, then leave it over the winter. By next spring the worms will, hopefully, have worked their magic, though you can lightly fork it in then if it's still clumpy. If you opt for the no-dig approach, you have the added bonus of using the compost layer as a mulch before the worms get to work. This will keep weeds down and moisture in – as well as saving you from a bad 'digging' back and blisters! The no-dig approach also means that you can actively improve your soil without damaging the roots of existing plants as you thrust in the spade. In my opinion, albeit very biased, this makes the choice between the dig and no-dig options a real no-brainer.

Heavy clay soils do, however, need a bit more attention: worms may draw organic matter from the surface and incorporate it into the soil, but they will not do the same with the grit or horticultural sand that are vital to improving drainage. The good thing is that you need to dig in the grit only once and it is there for life, so an hour or two of manual labour should transform your soil forever. You could theoretically do this at any time of year, but I reckon the best time to do this is autumn in order to prevent damage to the roots or shoots of plants that are actively growing.

Annuals and perennials

This is a bit of geeky, but really important, gardening terminology describing the lifespan of a plant – and thus determining how often you'll need to plant it. An annual plant, as its name suggests, grows from seed, flowers, sets seed and dies all in one year. A perennial grows, flowers and sets seed year after year without dying. ('Biennials' such as mullein, meanwhile, have a lifespan of two years. Growing from seed one year, then flowering, setting seed and dying the next.)

In general, perennials can be a little less work, as you do not have to sow them from seed each year. Instead, they keep growing year after year. Having said that, there are many annuals, such as sunflowers or borage, which happily sow their own seeds around your garden. This may create a lovely naturalistic effect or end up being a nightmare when they pop up everywhere! A little judicious weeding is needed where space is at a premium, but you can always pot up the seedlings and share them with friends. Perennials, meanwhile, form larger clumps each year, which can be divided and moved in autumn or winter to increase plant numbers.

Organic fertilizers

Fear over the potentially harmful effects of chemical fertilizers has created a huge interest in organic fertilizers in recent years. To my mind, the benefits of organic fertilizers stretch far beyond avoiding chemical residues, though.

While you can buy pelleted organic chicken manure and seaweed fertilizers in almost every garden centre these days, why not go down the no-cost route by picking up well-rotted manure from a local farmer or stables? Both are often more than happy to get rid of the stuff. You can even make your own organic fertilizer by starting a compost heap or bagging up leaf mould in big black bin bags (leave for a year or more to rot completely). Many local councils offer free compost when using council recycling schemes. (You drop off some cans or bottles for recycling and get bags of free compost in exchange – now that's a good deal!) If you live near the coast, you can scatter pieces of seaweed, collected from coastal walks, over the surface of your soil too; just be sure to rinse them first to wash of any salty residue, which could damage the plants. With so many organic fertilizers often being free to make and source, not to mention easier to apply (you don't have to calculate dilution rates, for example) and often more eco-friendly, what reason is there for not giving them a go?

Maintenance

If you are picking leaves regularly for use in remedies, there is little other maintenance required, apart from an occasional watering and a bit of weeding to keep things in check. Once your medicinal garden gets properly established, it'll need a spring tidy-up. I always think it's best to leave any cutting back of perennial plants until the following spring – that way, you'll have collected all the autumn seeds you need, the birds will have eaten the rest and you'll enjoy seeing the frost-covered stems during the long, cold days of winter.

IDENTIFYING YOUR PERSONAL AILMENT NEEDS

Plants are marvellous things – they can soothe an irritated stomach, headache or skin problems; aid digestion or circulation; minimize cold symptoms; and even boost the immune system. But when you're feeling under the weather, you need to know which plants to turn to for fast relief. What should you be using if you're prone to colds and flu, suffer from eczema or dermatitis or regularly get indigestion?

In the short term, you can buy all the plants in this book fresh or dried from herbal suppliers, health or Asian food shops or supermarkets (see Stockists, page 215). But in the long term it's much cheaper (and more fun!) to go down the self-sufficiency route and grow your own. Here's our list of the most outstanding plant performers you can buy and grow for various common ailments. Stock up on these and you'll have a natural medicine cabinet that'll help keep you and your family healthy all year round.

For digestive problems

For tummy complaints and digestive problems, try angelica, caraway seeds, ginger, fennel, marshmallow, peppermint and slippery elm, all wonderful stomach soothers.

What to grow: angelica (*Angelica archangelica*) and marshmallow are easy to grow in the garden. Ginger will root in a pot on your windowsill, though growing it to harvest is something of an experiment. Don't be disappointed if the root you unearth in autumn isn't very large – in a sunny year, you'll still be rewarded with architectural leaves and perhaps some exotic-looking flowers, and with patience you'll be able to harvest a good chunk of root from a mature plant. Caraway and fennel like sunny sites (harvest seeds in late summer/autumn); and peppermint likes a bit of shade – all the mints are best grown in pots, as they can be invasive.

What to buy: slippery elm powder (not capsules), dried angelica and marshmallow root from herbal suppliers and health food shops. Ginger, fennel and caraway seeds from Asian food shops or supermarkets.

For respiratory problems

To wage war on colds and flu this winter, stock up on echinacea, elderberries, eucalyptus, ginger, goji berries, nettles, onions and garlic.

What to grow: pick elderberries, goji berries (both in early autumn), and nettles in the wild (or you can plant them if you really want!). Find a eucalyptus tree in your neighbourhood and ask for a few leaves. Echinacea, garlic and onions grow well outside. For ginger, see above.

What to buy: onions, garlic and ginger from greengrocers. Dried elderberries, eucalyptus leaves, nettles, echinacea root or tincture from herbal specialists or health food shops. Dried goji berries from Asian food shops (where they can be as little as half the price of those in fancy health food stores).

For dermatological problems

To soothe skin problems including cuts, rashes, bruises, burns, insect bites, itchiness, eczema and psoriasis, keep the following handy: aloe vera, chamomile, chickweed, pot marigold, plantain, St John's wort, tea tree and witch hazel.

What to grow: chickweed and plantain grow prolifically in the wild (and the latter perhaps in your lawn too!). Aloe vera will grow in a pot; cut off a leaf whenever you need one. Chamomile and pot marigold (*Calendula officinalis*) like a sunny border (or pot), and St John's wort will be happy in partial shade; harvest the flowering tops as they bloom in early summer. Witch hazel (*Hamamelis virginiana*) flowers in winter, but you can use the twigs and leaves throughout the year. It will tolerate most conditions: sun, part shade or a deeper shady woodland setting.

What to buy: tea tree essential oil, dried chamomile, dried marigold flowers, dried St John's wort and aloe vera gel from herbal suppliers and health food shops. Distilled witch hazel is handy for everyday use, from pharmacies.

For kids

In their remedies, children like plants that look and taste sweet and fruity, such as bilberries, blackberries, blackcurrants, chamomile, elderberries, honeysuckle, mint, rosehip — oh, and ginger is great for travel sickness.

What to grow: you can pick elderberries, blackberries and rosehips from wild hedgerows in late summer/early autumn. Mint (all varieties) grows well in pots in semi-shade. For ginger, see above. Blackcurrant and bilberry bushes need space; you can grow both in pots. Honeysuckle grows wild, in the garden or in a large pot with support. Chamomile likes sun, preferably in a border, though pots will do.

What to buy: bilberries, blackcurrants, blackberries, ginger and fresh mint from greengrocers or supermarkets. Dried chamomile, elderberries and rosehips from herbal suppliers and health food shops.

For muscular & joint problems

To soothe sore muscles and bring topical relief to stiff joints, keep a good supply of chilli, eucalyptus, ginger, horseradish, liquorice and turmeric.

What to grow: horseradish, turmeric. Chilli is surprisingly high yielding; one plant will keep you in chillies almost all year round and you can save and sow the seeds from your own fruit. Ginger (see above). All four can be grown in pots.

Liquorice in pots or the border. Eucalyptus trees are huge – look for one in the neighbourhood and ask for some leaves if you don't have room to plant your own, although some eucalyptus, such as *eucalyptus gunnii,* can be pruned or cut right back so space need not be a problem.

What to buy: chilli peppers, ginger, horseradish root, liquorice root, turmeric root or powder from Asian or ethnic food shops, greengrocers and supermarkets. Dried eucalyptus leaves from herbal suppliers.

For emotional problems

What to grow: gotu kola, lemon balm, St John's wort and vervain grow easily in the garden, though gotu kola and vervain are tender, so bring under cover in winter. (See how to plant a Raise the Spirits pot on page 170.) Rose root actually likes the cold, but give it good drainage; it's a succulent plant and you don't want it to rot through a wet winter. Ginseng (*Panax ginseng*) grows well here, but roots from 6–7-year-old plants are used, so it may be easier to buy!

What to buy: *Panax ginseng* roots from Asian and health food shops. Dried gotu kola, St John's wort and vervain from herbal suppliers.

For hormonal problems

What to grow: raspberry bushes need a bit of space, but can be grown in a large pot. Sage will grow in pots or in the garden.

What to buy: dried raspberry leaves from herbal suppliers, fresh sage from supermarkets.

For headaches

What to grow: rosemary and feverfew are easily cultivated in the garden. Feverfew is great value too because it'll self-seed like crazy, and you'll always have it once you've planted it. Willow (*Salix spp.*) grows along riverbanks – ask permission from your local authority if you want to harvest a little of the inner bark from young branches in spring.

What to buy: willow bark and dried feverfew leaves from herbal suppliers, fresh rosemary from supermarkets.

MAKING

BASIC REMEDY SKILLS

Creating remedies is just like cooking. In fact, it can often be much easier – there are no tricky risottos, white sauces or soufflés, for a start.

There are only two basic methods of extracting the essential ingredients of plants at home: by steeping them in a cold liquid (oil, vinegar, alcohol, glycerine, honey); or by heating them in a warm liquid (water or syrup – a mixture of water and sugar). These plant extracts can be applied to the body externally in the form of salves, rubs, bath and body scrubs, mouthwashes, face masks and moisturizing creams, or internally as drinks, soups, cough syrups, lozenges, lovely old-fashioned tonics, jellies and lollies, and even apéritifs and cocktails.

Some methods are more suitable than others for preparing certain herbs – it depends on the nature of the active ingredients they contain. All the methods in these recipes are specially designed to deliver the active ingredients in the optimum way.

Before you start, read this simple introduction to the best ways of extracting plant ingredients, plus a couple of basic remedy-making skills you'll find useful. Then you can get cracking...

Infusions

There's nothing easier than making a cup of tea with your plants – just put them in a teapot and pour freshly boiled water over. This is called an infusion, and it's definitely the quickest way to take in the goodness of plants (apart from those you can eat raw in salads!).

To make an infusion: you'll need about 30g fresh or 15g dried leaves or flowers for every 500ml of water. If you don't have a teapot, use a glass bowl, but make sure you put a cover over it (a large plate will do), so the essential oils don't evaporate. Leave the tea to steep for about 8–10 minutes, then strain and drink. Infusions are also used in the making of creams and lotions, and you can pour them into your bath for a soothing soak. Use this infusion method for flowers and leaves. You can add a little honey or sugar if you have a sweet tooth.

Storage Teas are best drunk the same day, but you can make up a batch of 3 cups in the morning, store covered in the refrigerator, then reheat as needed.

Decoctions

A decoction is just like a tea, but with plants left to simmer for a while – tougher plant materials like roots, twigs, seeds and bark need a longer cooking time to extract their essential ingredients.

To make a decoction: wash and cut up the roots, twigs or bark to expose a large surface area and make the extraction easier. In a pan, put about 30g chopped fresh plant material (or 15g dried) for every 500ml of water. Cover the pan, bring to the boil, then simmer for at least 10 minutes (and up to 30 minutes for tougher roots). Strain before drinking. Decoctions are also used in making lotions and creams, and you can pour them liberally into the bath.

Storage Best drunk the same day. But, as with infusions, you can make up a batch of 3 cups in the morning, store covered in the refrigerator, then reheat as needed to drink throughout the day.

Infused oils

Infused oils capture the flavour, colour and perfume as well as the essential, health-giving compounds of plants. They're ideal for use as massage and bath oils, and as a base from which to make creams, rubs and salves. Herb oils like basil, rosemary and thyme can also be used in cooking or salad dressings. You can make single-flavour oils or blend two or more plants together to make a mixed-flavour oil – these are also great as homemade gifts.

To make an infused oil: three-quarters fill a clean glass, screw-top or Kilner jar with plant material, crushing lightly to release the essential compounds. Pour over the oil of your choice (see below), making sure all the plants are completely submerged – stray leaves or flowers can go mouldy and affect oil quality.

Storage Seal, and leave in a warm, sunny spot for 2 weeks, shaking the bottle every couple of days, and pushing down any uncovered plant material. Strain into a sterilized bottle.

Choosing base oils

The base oil you choose depends on how you're going to be using the infused oil. If it's for creams and lotions, choose a light, non-greasy vegetable oil such as sunflower, safflower, palm or grapeseed oil – my favourite is sunflower oil because it is the cheapest and most readily available. Who would have thought the same stuff you fry your chips in would turn out to be the best for making luxurious creams and bath products? For very dry skin, however, heavier oils such as olive, avocado or wheatgerm are excellent, though a little more pricey. If it's for internal use, choose an oil you like to cook with – for example, sunflower, sesame, groundnut, walnut or olive oil. Oils can go rancid if stored badly, so check it's okay (just taste a little) before you use it.

Quick solution! If you need an infused oil for a recipe and don't have 2 weeks to spare, try this fast maceration instead. Put the plant material in a glass bowl, cover with oil, then place above a pan of boiling water and cook, covered, for 20 minutes to 1 hour, or until the oil has taken on the colour and flavour of the herbs. Strain and bottle.

Storage Infused oils will last for 6 months to 1 year if stored in a cool, dark place.

Vinegars

You can infuse vinegars with fresh plant material in exactly the same way as oils. They are very palatable as cordials sweetened with honey, and as daily tonics taken by the spoonful. They work well in compresses, as gargles and mouthwashes, to add shine to hair in rinses or just poured into the bath to soothe skin. They also add an extra depth of flavour in cooking and salad dressings

To make an infused vinegar: three-quarters fill a clean Kilner jar with plant material, crushing lightly to help release the essential compounds. Pour over cider or white wine vinegar to cover (don't use malt), making sure the plants are completely submerged.

Storage Seal, and leave in a warm, sunny spot for 2 weeks, shaking the bottle every couple of days, and pushing down any uncovered plant material. When ready, strain and pour into a sterilized bottle.

Tinctures

When you use alcohol to extract the active ingredients from plants, it's called a tincture. Alcohol is more effective than oil and vinegar at extraction from tough plant material such as roots and resins. It's also a good preservative, so tinctures last longer than other preparations, and as they are more concentrated, you use less. These recipes mostly specify vodka because it is colourless and almost tasteless, which allows the flavour of the plants to come through. But whisky, brandy, gin or rum are just as effective – any distilled alcohol can be used as long as it is at least 80% proof (ie 40% alcohol). If made with concentrations below that, tinctures will deteriorate more quickly.

Tinctures are very handy – they're easy to store, and give you concentrated plant goodness whenever you need it. They're usually taken a teaspoonful a day when required, and they work fast, being absorbed quickly into the bloodstream. If you don't want to take alcoholic tinctures, an alternative is a glycerite.

To make a tincture: three-quarters fill a small Kilner or glass jar with plant material, then cover with the alcohol of your choice, making sure all the plants are completely submerged. Seal, and leave in a dark place at room temperature for between 8 days to 1 month (the length of time depends on the 'toughness' of the plant material – resins and roots take longer than flowers and leaves). Shake the bottle occasionally, making sure all plant material remains covered. When ready, strain into small, dark glass bottles.

Storage Using amber, black or blue glass will help preserve the tincture longer. Kept in a cool, dark place, tinctures will last for 2 years (and sometimes longer).

Glycerites

If you don't want to use alcohol, you can extract the active constituents in plants with glycerine instead. Glycerine is a pure substance, like sugar or salt, which tastes sweet and syrupy, so it is often used in children's remedies as a cordial to which you add water. It's also soothing and emollient, and is good for skin preparations and sore throat and cough preparations, as well as for calming the digestive system. Glycerine is not as efficient as alcohol at extracting essential plant compounds, so the end result is less concentrated and has a shorter shelf life.

To make a basic glycerite: three-quarters fill a Kilner or other glass jar with plant material (leaves and flowers are best), crushing lightly to help release the essential compounds. Pour glycerine over to cover, making sure all the plants are completely submerged. Seal, and leave on a warm, bright windowsill for 2 weeks to infuse, shaking every couple of days. Strain into bottles.

Storage Glycerites will keep for up to 1 year.

Gels

Gels are used medicinally as jellies and in skin preparations – they have good astringent or skin-tightening properties – and also in many cosmetics including hair and aftershave gels and face masks. The gel-like consistency is achieved by adding gelatine, or other clear thickener such as xanthan gum, to the recipe at the appropriate time, then whisking with or without heat until the mixture thickens and a gel is formed. I usually use powdered vegetable gelatine, which dissolves easily and has good thickening properties – you can buy it from the baking section of most supermarkets.

To make a simple face mask gel: in a pan, pour 100ml of a plant-based infusion of your choice. Dissolve a sachet of vegetable gelatine into the infusion (usually one 6g sachet per 100ml liquid, but it depends on the brand you buy – I always make it 3 times stronger than advised on the packet). Stir to dissolve, then heat gently for a couple of minutes, whisking vigorously until you get a smooth gel. If you like, whisk in a few drops of an essential oil of your choice for its medicinal properties or scent.

Storage Gelatine-based remedies don't keep well. Store in the refrigerator and use within 2 days if taking internally. Cosmetic and hair gels will keep in the refrigerator for up to 4 weeks.

Ointments, salves & balms

Ointments, salves and medicinal balms are all oil and wax preparations, made to various consistencies. An ointment is thinner than a salve, and is usually applied over large areas of the body to soothe skin, or to rub into the chest as an expectorant. Salves and medicinal balms are thicker and waxier, and tend to be used on specific areas such as joints (or lips!). All are easy to make, by heating an emulsifier such as beeswax or emulsifying wax with an infused oil – you simply add more emulsifier to make a thicker salve or less for a thinner ointment.

To make a basic ointment: in a glass bowl, put 300ml of an infused oil with 25g beeswax. (Use granules, or break solid wax into small pieces – you can even use 100% beeswax candles.) Stand the bowl over a pan of simmering water, and stir gently until all the wax has melted. Pour while still warm into wide-mouthed salve jars – the ointment thickens as it cools.

Getting the right consistency: To check if the ointment is the consistency you want, drop a little into a glass of iced water – if it turns into a ball, it'll be a thick balm; if it disperses on the surface, you'll have the consistency of a thinner ointment. To make the mixture thicker, add an extra ½ teaspoon of beeswax at a time; to make it thinner, add 1 extra teaspoon of infused oil at a time. Heat again and re-test until you're happy with it.

Storage Ointments, salves and balms will keep for 1 year.

Creams

Creams are an excellent way to apply plants' active compounds to skin, being quickly absorbed and moisturizing. They're also great fun to make, and much more cost-effective than buying in a shop. A cream is basically a mixture of water and oil, held together with an emulsifier. I tend to use a combination of beeswax and emulsifying wax. It's true that creams are just a little trickier to make than salves, but if you follow a few simple rules, you'll soon pick up the knack.

To make a basic cream: put 40ml infused oil in a glass bowl with 6 teaspoons of emulsifying wax and 2 teaspoons of beeswax. Heat the bowl over a pan of simmering water, stirring occasionally, until the wax is completely dissolved. Then it's like making mayonnaise. Pour in 250ml warm water in a thin, steady stream, while whisking vigorously. Whisk for about 5 minutes, scraping the sides of the bowl if necessary, until the mixture forms an emulsion. Take the pan off the heat and keep whisking while the cream cools and thickens, to stop the oil and water separating. You can whisk in a few drops of an essential oil while the cream is cooling, to add medicinal qualities and scent. Essential oils even act as a natural preservative, because of their anti-microbial properties. Then spoon the cream into a sterile wide-mouthed jar and seal. (For very simple instructions on how to sterilize jars, see below.)

Storage Creams last for up to 2 months in the refrigerator.

Getting creams right... These guidelines will help your creams come out successfully:

» Make sure both liquids are at approximately the same temperature (about 70°C or slightly higher) before you start mixing – an even emulsion is less likely to occur if one is much hotter or colder.

» Dribble the infusion into the oil very slowly – if you blob too much in at a time, it won't emulsify well.

» Keep beating during the cooling process to get a good consistency. The cream thickens as it cools.

» Be patient! The cream will thicken upon cooling, so don't be disheartened if you have a smooth, white liquid that is a little runny. It will thicken up greatly as soon as it cools to room temperature.

Sterilizing bottles and jars

Before you use any glass bottles and jars for storing your remedies, quickly sterilize them. I always put them through the hottest spin of the dishwasher and leave them to dry in the steam. But you can also wash them in very hot soapy water, then stand them upside down on some newspaper, and place in the oven at a low setting (about 70ºC) for about 20 minutes. Then they're ready for filling.

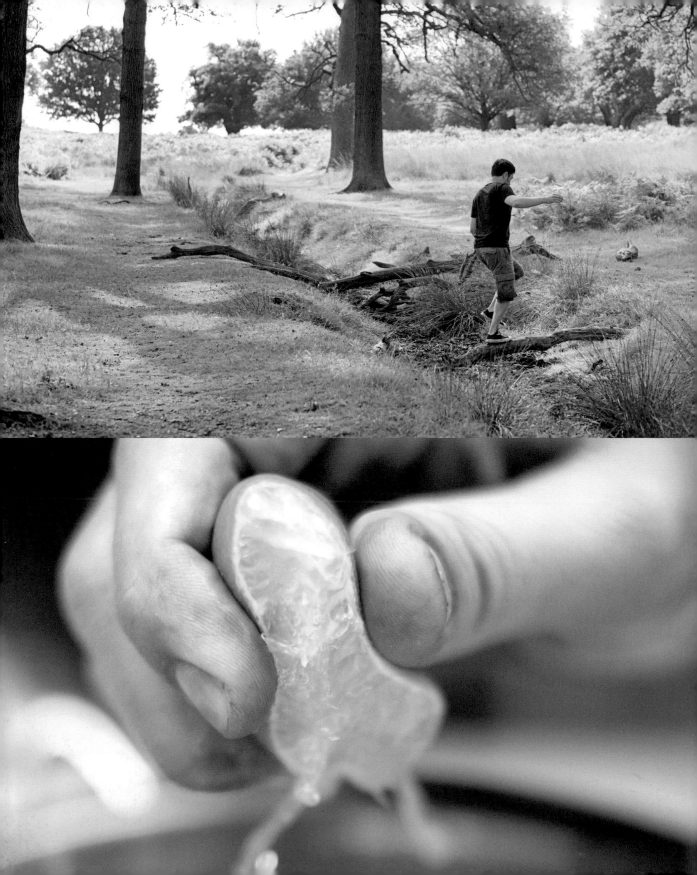

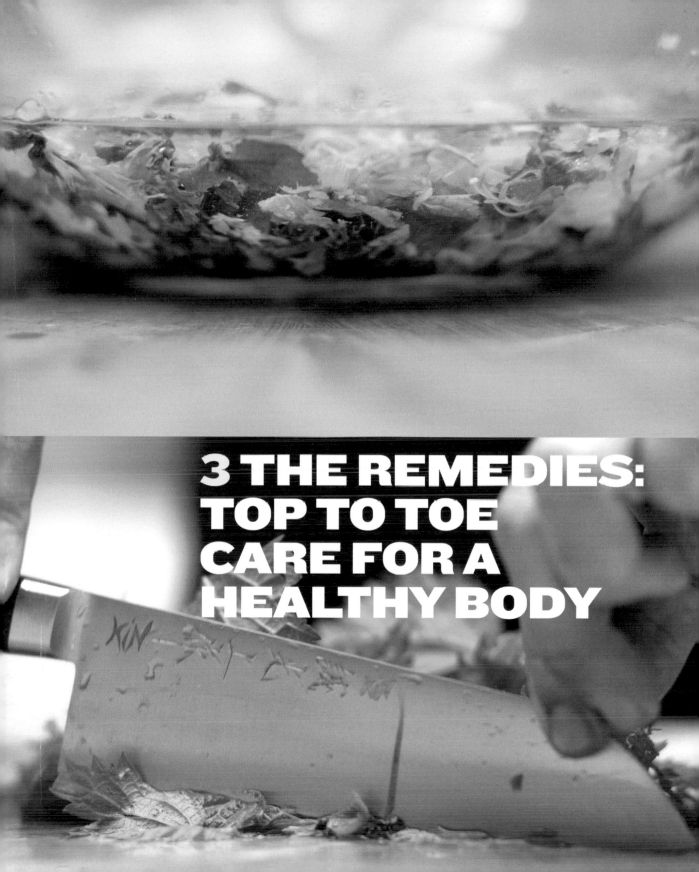

3 THE REMEDIES: TOP TO TOE CARE FOR A HEALTHY BODY

REMEDIES

Herbal remedies can have a reputation for being rather ominous, dark brews, laboriously boiled for hours and knocked back in a single traumatic gulp, with your fingers firmly pinched over your nose.

Despite my best efforts to avoid the issue, I must confess that for many old-school traditional remedies this reputation is well deserved. I was subjected to a fair few acrid concoctions when growing up, and can personally confirm their powerful pre-emptive placebo effect. Nothing can make a sick child's symptoms miraculously disappear as fast as being presented with a murky bowl of soup scattered with unidentified roots and twigs. Sorry, Mum.

Luckily, not all natural medicines have to be this way, and I am a passionate believer (almost evangelical, in fact) that the vast majority are unbelievably easy to make and can look and taste truly wonderful.

What I find incredibly exciting from a culinary perspective is that herbal remedies can open up a whole range of truly amazing flavours to which we would otherwise be oblivious. Meadowsweet blossoms, traditionally used to relieve pain, have a fizzy, sweet flavour of rich marzipan and elderflowers, while echinacea has an almost electric, metallic tingle, provided by alkylamides (the group of chemicals that give the plant its immune-enhancing effects). I know how geeky this sounds, but I am convinced that the weird and wonderful flavours of many medicinal plants are perfect for chefs and mixologists. You just wait, it won't be long before feverfew martinis are on the menus of swanky cocktail bars everywhere. But I digress.

Experimenting in my kitchen at home with all sorts of medicinal ingredients for this book, I have created a collection of entirely new recipes. These are my modern twist on age-old remedies and are as easy to make as they are delicious to drink, wonderful to smell and soothing to apply. The intensely bitter, drying taste of willow bark tea (one of the substances from which aspirin was first derived) has been turned into a smoky, sweet willow and lime granita, a modern (and, frankly, far more palatable) take on the original, which nevertheless does just as good a job. True, my experiments don't always work out right, and some recipes have undergone over a dozen reformulations before I finally got them spot on, but I think that's half the fun. There are fewer hard and fast rules with herbal remedies than you might imagine; as long as you pick the right plant and prepare it in a broadly similar way to its traditional use and dosage, there is plenty of room to mix and match and play around.

I suppose the useful thing is that most of the laborious trial-and-error work has been done by me, leaving you with a collection of tried-and-tested modern home remedies. They are presented here more or less according to the part of the body they are used to treat, to give you a top-to-toe guide to natural medicines that can easily be prepared at home. All you have to do now is get stuck in!

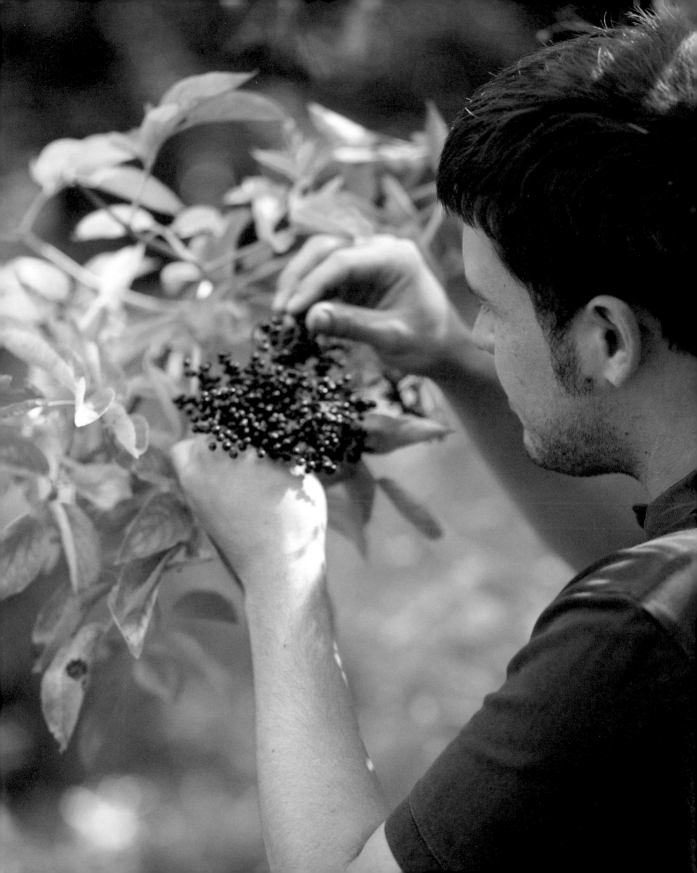

DERMATOLOGICAL

Soothing botanical creams, salves and balms to help take the heat out of irritated skin, reduce inflammation and accelerate healing – and leave skin feeling soft and moisturized too.

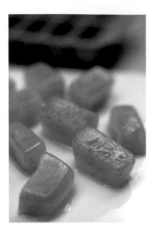

Aloe Vera and Marigold Frozen Gel Cubes for Burns

Aloe vera is without doubt the ultimate instant skin soother. You can simply snap off one of its squidgy gel-packed leaves, which work like living first-aid sachets, and apply it directly to the skin – no fuss necessary. But nature can be improved upon. These ice-cold aloe and marigold gel cubes are especially cooling for sunburned skin, helping to prevent scarring, inflammation and infection and to promote healing – though they can be used on any kind of burn.

2 mature fresh
aloe vera leaves

4 fresh marigold flower
heads
(*Calendula officinalis*)

16 drops lavender
essential oil
(I drop per ice cube)

I Peel the fresh aloe leaves (see Tip below) to give you a gooey mass of gel.

2 Put into a blender with the marigold flowers and whizz until smooth.

3 Pour the gel into ice-cube trays, adding a drop of lavender essential oil into each individual cube. Freeze until solid.

USE Apply a cube directly to the affected area as needed. The ice cubes melt quickly to produce masses of fragrant soothing gel. Don't forget to have a paper towel or cloth handy to mop up the melted gel; the goo has a habit of going everywhere!

STORAGE Will keep in the freezer for up to 6 months.

james's tip To peel an aloe leaf: cut a mature leaf from the outside of the plant, as close to the base as you can (you can store these leaves in the refrigerator for 2 weeks; amazingly, they 'seal' themselves at the cut edges). Slice off the ends, trimming the spikes off the sides with a sharp knife. Then place the aloe flat on the chopping board and run the knife inside the skin, slicing it off as you would skin a fish – be careful, the gel is very slippery and your knife can slide all over the place. Turn and repeat, taking off the skin on the other side. You're left with a gooey mass of slippery gel, and you can pop this straight into the blender.

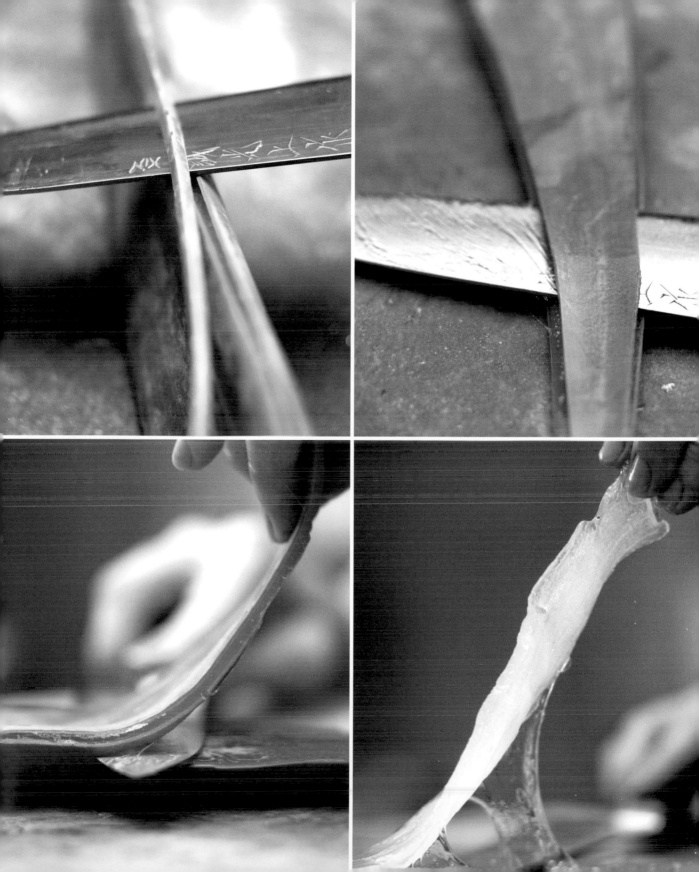

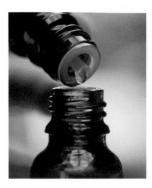

A Simple Cream

This is an incredibly simple recipe for a basic cream. Once you have mastered this, and trust me it isn't rocket science, you can adapt it to your own needs by mixing and matching it with other ingredients.

250ml warm water (you could swap this for any herbal decoction or infusion you like)

2 tsp beeswax

6 tsp emulsifying wax

40ml sunflower oil (you can experiment with other oils such as almond, olive, etc, or even use oils infused with herbs)

2 tsp vitamin C powder (optional)

6-12 drops whichever essential oil takes your fancy (optional)

1 Combine the beeswax, emulsifying wax and oil together in a pan and heat very gently until the waxes fully dissolve.

2 Pour the warm water in a thin stream into the oil and wax mixture, whisking vigorously all the time. You should see an instant colour change as the mix turns creamy white. Don't panic however if it looks a little thin textured, this will thicken significantly as it cools. Although very simple to get right, this is the single most important stage of making a cream. If you simply bung in all the water in one go, or don't whisk the mixture well enough as you are adding it, the two liquids will not combine to form the smooth emulsion you are looking for. Slow pouring and vigorous whisking are key.

3 Stir in the vitamin C powder (which acts as a natural preservative) and essential oils if desired, and bottle up in clean screw-top jars.

USE Apply the cream liberally wherever you feel the need.

STORAGE Will keep in the fridge for up to 1 month.

james's tip I always liken making creams to the ordering a drink at high-street coffee chains, where you can have your latte non-fat, with an extra shot of espresso, a dash of hazelnut syrup, despite us all knowing it's basically just coffee. Well in the same way you could add a couple of drops of whichever essential oil you fancy to adapt its smell, infuse either the water or oil component (or both) with herbs to give it an extra kick, and even try out different base oils – the sky is the limit!

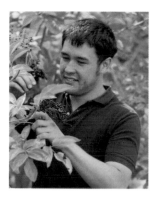

Elder and Neem Insect Repellent Gel

This all-natural mozzy repellent conveniently doubles up as a cooling, anti-inflammatory 'aftersun' gel. Sweet and spicy, the combination of savoury neem and lemony citronella makes it smell miles better than anything you can get over the counter. Glycerine is available in most pharmacies, and can usually be found among the cough syrups. Neem oil and citronella essential oil can both be bought from health food shops.

8 heaped tbsp fresh elder leaves and buds

about 100ml glycerine

50ml neem oil

4ml citronella essential oil

100g aloe vera gel

1 Rinse the elder leaves and buds in running water. Pat dry with a paper towel, then bruise with a pestle and mortar or rolling pin. Place in a clean, sealable glass jar, then pour on enough glycerine to cover the plant material and close the jar. Leave for 2 weeks, shaking occasionally. Strain through muslin. The resultant liquid is known as a glycerite (basically an infused glycerine), and is one of the easiest ways to extract the best out of a whole range of herbs.

2 In another bowl, add the neem oil to the citronella essential oil and stir. Pour in 50ml of the elder leaf glycerite and whisk together thoroughly to make a gel. Finally, stir in the aloe vera gel and pour into a 300ml bottle.

USE Massage the gel into the skin, especially exposed areas like ankles, wrists and neck, avoiding the eyes. Cover the whole body and remember to re-apply after washing or bathing in the evening or at night. A little goes a long way since it's quite strong.

CAUTION If any irritation occurs, wash off at once.

STORAGE Will keep for up to 1 year in a cool, dark place.

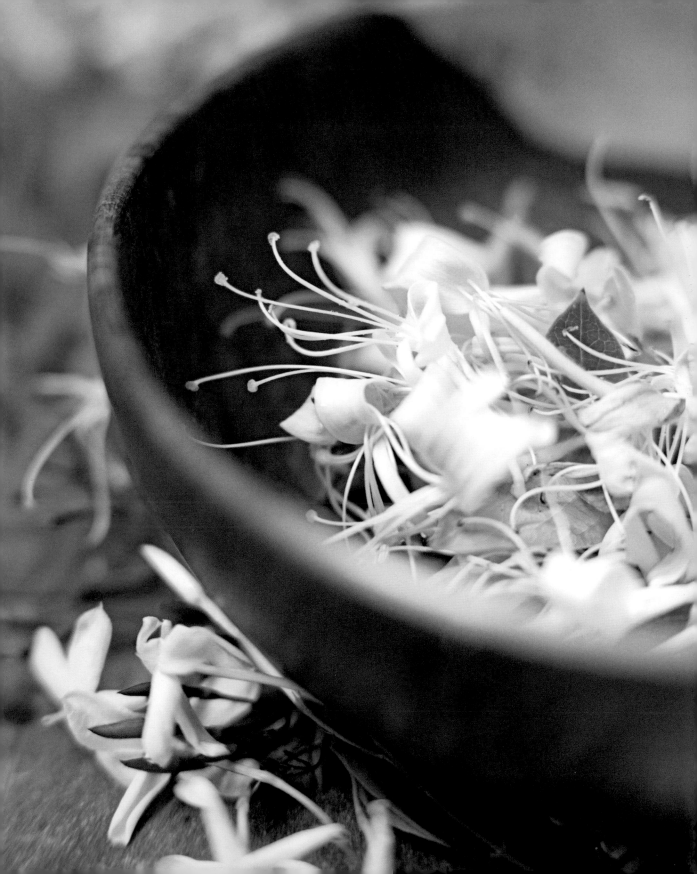

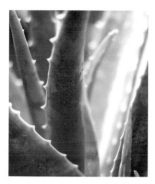

Aloe and Slippery Elm Antiseptic Poultice

This is an indispensable item of the homemade first-aid kit – an antiseptic 'drawing' poultice to help treat infected cuts, skin ulcers, boils, bites and stings. Its team of botanical ingredients can help draw out poisons, reduce inflammation and pain, and accelerate healing.

10g slippery elm powder

20g manuka honey

18ml aloe vera juice

4ml lavender
essential oil

Mix all the ingredients together in a clean screw-top jar.

USE Clean and dry the affected area, apply the paste, then cover with a plaster and/or bandages. Change the dressing every 12 hours.

STORAGE Keeps for up to 1 year in an airtight jar.

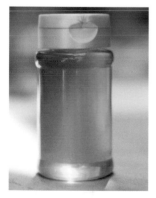

Manuka Honey Wound Healer

The antiseptic powers of manuka honey have been used for centuries by the Maori people in its native New Zealand to draw out infections. By teaming it with lavender, another potent antiseptic, you get a simple and effective salve to aid the healing of wounds, from infected cuts to ulcers.

1 jar manuka honey

2 drops lavender
essential oil

sterile wound dressing

USE Clean and dry the wound, ensuring no foreign objects are present. Mix the honey and essential oil together and apply the fragrant mix directly to the wound. Dress the wound with a sterile dressing.

Change the dressing daily, twice daily if necessary. When changing the dressing, it is important that you wash the wound with sterile water (or boiled and cooled water) or saline solution. Reapply the honey mix before redressing.

Herb Robert Cream

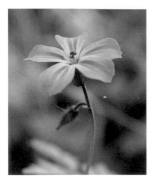

Herb Robert is a dainty wild geranium that grows freely in gardens and the countryside, often as a common weed. It was traditionally used as a cure-all and this gentle cream can help soothe a variety of skin conditions, including bruises, thread veins and chilblains. It's also worth trying for varicose veins. Compound benzoin tincture is also known, rather exotically, as friar's balsam. See page 212.

To make the plant juice:
- 4–5 handfuls fresh herb Robert (about 6–8 whole plants)
- 2–6 sprigs fresh rosemary, each about 15–20cm long
- 8 tsp manuka honey

To make the cream:
- 16g beeswax
- 8g emulsifying wax
- 80ml olive oil
- 6 drops benzoin or compound benzoin tincture

1 Place the herb Robert and rosemary in a large mortar with the manuka honey, and pound to a paste. Allow to sit for 10 minutes while the sugar in the honey draws the active ingredients out of the plants. Place the sweet paste in clean muslin and squeeze out the juice into a small bowl.

2 Take 1½ tablespoons of the sweetened juice and put into a small pan. Heat quickly until it steams but doesn't boil, then turn off the heat immediately. This process greatly increases its shelf life.

3 Melt the waxes in the olive oil in a glass heatproof bowl over a pan of boiling water, then remove from the heat. Pour the warmed plant juice into the bowl with the melted waxes and oil, then add the compound benzoin tincture and whisk together. Continue whisking while it cools slightly to stop ingredients separating, then put in a wide-mouthed jar and refrigerate.

USE Apply to affected area 3–4 times a day as needed.

STORAGE Will keep for up to 3 months in the refrigerator.

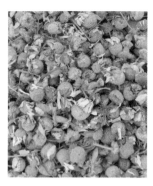

Oat and Chamomile Bath Bag for Eczema

A soothing bath treat that will help soften and moisturize all skin types, though it's particularly useful for dermatitis, eczema and other irritated, itchy skin conditions.

8 tbsp oats

3g dried chamomile flowers

Cut a 25–30cm square of muslin and lay flat. In a bowl, mix the oats and chamomile flowers together. Tip into the middle of the muslin. Gather the corners of the muslin and secure into a ball with string.

USE Run a full bath, climb in, and soak the bag in the water for a few minutes. Then rub the bag directly on your skin as a gentle exfoliator – avoid damaged skin if using for eczema. Once finished, drop the ball into the bath and squeeze (the water will look a little milky). Remain in the bath for a further 10 minutes. Use twice weekly to treat eczema.

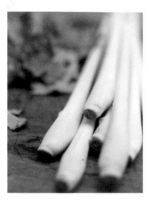

Lemongrass Insect Repellent

Fresh lemongrass is easier to find than fresh citronella grass (which you can buy only from specialist nurseries). It works in a similar way as a potent natural insect repellent, with the added benefit of antibacterial and antifungal properties. Here, I've mixed it with a couple of other aromatic insecticidal plants for a modern take on a traditional South-East Asian bug-repellent oil, with a sweet spicy fragrance that smells wonderful to anyone but insects.

10 lemongrass sticks

4 tsp scented pelargonium 'Citronella' leaves (about 15 leaves)

4 tsp whole cloves

400ml sunflower oil, to cover

1 Wash and chop the lemongrass sticks and pelargonium leaves, and place both in a blender with the cloves. Add the oil, then whizz until pulped.

2 Place the pulp in a glass heatproof bowl and cover. Put the bowl over a pan of boiling water on a low heat, making sure there are no gaps around the bowl, and leave for 1 hour. Keep checking that the pan does not boil dry.

3 Leave to cool, then strain the citrus- and spice-scented oil through muslin to remove all the fibrous bits, and store in a pump spray bottle.

USE Shake the bottle well, then spray liberally onto skin up to 4 times a day, paying particular attention to exposed areas like ankles, wrists and neck, and avoiding the eyes. Re-apply after washing or bathing, and before bed.

CAUTION If any irritation occurs, wash off immediately.

STORAGE Will keep for up to 1 year in a cool, dark place.

> **james's tip** Lemongrass makes a beautiful houseplant that's as fragrant as it is unusual, and the best thing is that planting one couldn't be easier. All you do is pop some fresh sticks (the fresher the better) into a glass of water with the fattest end down, and leave them on a sunny windowsill. (You can use lemongrass sticks bought at the supermarket.) In just a few weeks, the sticks will send out masses of tangled white and lemon-scented shoots, which can then be potted up in some well-drained compost. Keep in a sunny spot, water about once a week and you will be rewarded with a year-round supply of fresh, air-mile-free lemongrass.

DIGESTIVE

Teas, tablets and tonics to help soothe stomach and gastrointestinal upsets, and alleviate the symptoms of gas, bloating, heartburn, irritable bowel and other digestive complaints.

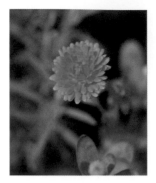

Wild Herb Tea for Soothing the Digestive Tract

You'll find all these plants growing wild (see foraging tips on page 208) or in gardens in summertime – pick and dry them then, so you can make up a good quantity of this tea to last you through autumn and winter.

15g marshmallow leaves, dried

10g plantain leaves (*Plantago major* or *P. lanceolata*), dried

15g marigold flowers (*Calendula officinalis*), dried

10g wild marjoram (*Origanum vulgare*) leaves, dried

Marshmallow plants are under threat in the wild, but the good news is they are incredibly easy to grow in any back garden. By planting them, you not only get a stunning garden plant and endless supplies of flowers and leaves for remedies, but you also do your bit to help conserve a threatened species.

1 Combine the dried herbs and store in an airtight container. This will make enough for about 5–6 cups of tea; if you want to make larger amounts, just multiply the quantities.

2 To make the tea, use 1–2 teaspoons per cup of boiling water. Cover and leave to infuse for 10 minutes, before straining and drinking.

USE Drink freely as needed.

CAUTION If pregnant, leave out the wild marjoram.

STORAGE The dried tea mix will keep in an airtight container for up to 1 year.

VARIATION FOR ACIDIC TUMMIES

This tea can help soothe acidic tummies, thanks to the meadowsweet: mix 10g German chamomile (*Matricaria recutita*) flowers, 10g lemon balm leaves, 15g meadowsweet flowers and 5g peppermint leaves. Follow the recipe above. This will make enough for about 3 cups of tea.

CAUTION If pregnant or allergic to aspirin, leave out the lemon balm and meadowsweet. Do not use with children under 16.

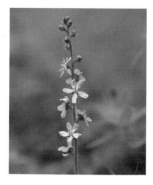

Marshmallow and Agrimony Ice Tea for Soothing the Digestive Tract

The combination of agrimony, long used to help relax a tense gut, and marshmallow, which soothes gastric inflammation, makes this a gentle remedy for irritable bowel and other digestive problems.

10g agrimony
(leaves and flowers)

300ml water,
freshly boiled

20g marshmallow root

runny honey to taste

1 Put the agrimony in a mug, pour over the water and leave to infuse, covered, until cool. Strain.

2 Pour the cold agrimony infusion over the marshmallow root (in a jug if making large amounts) and leave in the refrigerator overnight. The next morning, strain off the root and then the tea is ready to drink. If you wish to sweeten the tea, stir in a little runny honey until dissolved. Enough to make 2 mugs; keep in the refrigerator until needed.

USE Sip slowly throughout the day.

CAUTION Do not use to treat constipation, as agrimony can aggravate symptoms.

STORAGE Best made fresh.

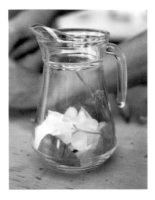

Angelica and Mint Cocktail for Indigestion

The inspiration here was to make aperitifs and digestifs fashionable again by packing as many stomach-soothing herbs into a hip, zingy cocktail that's more noughties' mojito than 70s' Drambuie. Angelica tastes wonderful and is traditionally used as a stomach-settler. You will find dried angelica root at any herbal supply shop. And the easiest way to get hold of chamomile flowers is from the supermarket: simply snip open a few chamomile tea bags.

For the tincture

100g fresh angelica root from the garden or 50g dried angelica root

25g fresh mint leaves

4 tsp fennel seeds

4 tsp dried German chamomile flowers (*Matricaria recutita*)

500ml vodka, or to cover

For the cocktail

sprig of mint

fresh dill leaves

lime slices

flat/uncarbonated ginger beer or ginger cordial (or other soft drink of your choice)

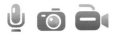

1 Wash and chop the angelica root and place in a glass jar with the fresh mint, fennel seeds and dried chamomile. Pour on the vodka to cover all the plant material. Seal the jar and leave to steep in a cold dark place for 10–14 days.

2 When ready, strain through muslin, reserving the liquid. This should produce about 400ml of vodka tincture.

3 Muddle a shot of the angelica tincture (about 35ml) with a sprig of mint, some dill leaves and lime slices in a tall glass. Top up with ice and flat or uncarbonated ginger beer or a soft cordial/drink you fancy.

NB You can make the drink considerably less alcoholic by adding the shot of tincture to boiling hot mixer/cordial, then allowing it to cool before adding the ice, mint, lime and dill. This works because the boiling hot mixer evaporates off most of the alcohol in the tincture.

USE Before meals to aid digestion or after meals if experiencing indigestion.

CAUTION Contains alcohol. Do not take if you are on medication from the doctor for a stomach ulcer or inflamed stomach lining – this is for simple indigestion and wind. Consideration should be taken when driving due to the alcohol content.

STORAGE Store the tincture in a cool, dark place for at least 1 year.

> **james's tip** I've used uncarbonated ginger beer here, just because I prefer the flavour of it, but if you're suffering from wind, try making it with carbonated instead. Believe it or not, the fizziness helps relieve trapped wind by encouraging the burp along…

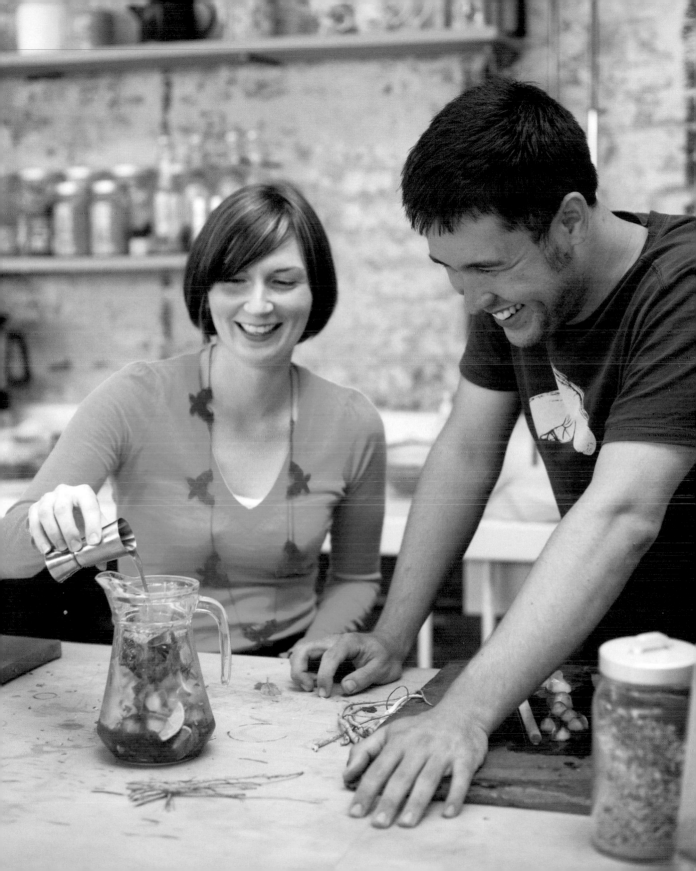

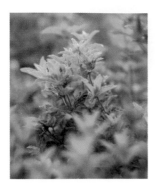

Peppermint Tummy Soother for Indigestion

Peppermint can help release trapped wind and soothe painful stomach griping. You can take this tonic by the spoonful or serve diluted as an after-dinner digestif cordial.

20g peppermint leaves

20g German chamomile flowers (*Matricaria recutita*) or 4 chamomile tea bags

900ml water

300g honey

75ml cider vinegar

1 Put the peppermint leaves and chamomile flowers in a pan and add the water, then cover and bring to the boil. Simmer gently for 15–20 minutes.

2 Leave to cool, then strain through a sieve into a measuring jug, pressing the plants with a spoon to get all the goodness out. Return the liquid to the pan and simmer gently, uncovered, until it has reduced down to 200ml. (Do this very slowly.)

3 Stir in the honey and vinegar and continue simmering for 20 minutes, or until thickened, but keep a close eye on it, as it can burn. Pour into a clean bottle.

USE For adults, take 2–3 teaspoons 3–6 times daily. Children over 2 years, take 1 teaspoon 3–6 times a day, when required. Or serve diluted, hot or cold, as a digestif cordial whenever needed.

STORAGE Will keep for 6 months in the refrigerator.

VARIATION FOR ACID REFLUX
For adults inclined to get acid reflux, replace the peppermint and chamomile with 40g meadowsweet flowers mixed with a small amount of rose petals, then follow the recipe above.

CAUTION Because of the meadowsweet, do not take if pregnant or if you're allergic to aspirin. Not suitable for children under 16.

'The remedy for me seems to have helped a lot. I found that before I'd get really bad stomach pains but now they're quite mild.' Aaliyah

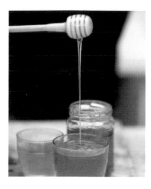

Slippery Elm Tablets for Acid Reflux or Gastritis

Slippery elm coats the mucous membranes of the oesophagus and acts as a protective barrier against stomach acids. Basically, it works like your body's own mucus to soothe inflamed and irritated tissues, a bit like a kind of prosthetic phlegm! Sweet and sticky, these tablets are far more palatable than my description makes them sound, I promise ... To find slippery elm powder, see Stockists on page 215.

2 heaped tbsp slippery elm powder

about 1–2 tsp honey

In a small bowl, mix the slippery elm powder with the honey until you get a thick paste (you may need to add a little more honey or powder). Roll the paste into small marble-sized balls. Dust each of them with a little more slippery elm powder, and store in an airtight jar.

USE Eat a tablet whenever experiencing digestive discomfort.

STORAGE Will keep up to 6 months in an airtight jar.

VARIATION MARSHMALLOW AND BISTORT BITES
Take 2 tbsp powdered marshmallow root and 1 tbsp powdered bistort (*Persicaria bistorta*) root – or use tormentil (*Potentilla erecta*) root instead. Mix to a paste with about 2–3 tsp honey (you may need a little more honey or powder to achieve the right consistency), then roll into marble-sized balls as above. Dust with a little more marshmallow root, then store in an airtight container for up to 6 months.

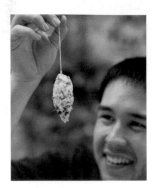

Fennel Sugar Mice for Flatulence

Sweet little sugar mice, reminiscent of childhood, but with peppermint and fennel seeds to help relieve bloating, soothe a windy stomach and give a subtle, sophisticated anise flavour. This makes 21 mice, and you can create them in any colour you like!

2 egg whites

250g icing sugar

200g dessicated coconut

4 tbsp fennel seeds

20 drops peppermint essential oil

a few drops homemade natural colourings (optional):

– for pink, use beetroot juice or blackberry jam

– for yellow, use turmeric

– for green, use juice pressed from chopped parsley

To decorate
cloves for eyes

pumpkin seeds for ears

string for tails

1 Beat the egg whites until frothy but not stiff. Stir in the sieved icing sugar, coconut, fennel seeds and peppermint essential oil, and mix until the mixture forms a firm dough. (Feel free to add more sugar if the mixture is not stiff enough to hold its shape.)

2 Knead in a few drops of colouring (optional).

3 Form the dough into 21 little mice shapes – greasing your hands lightly with sunflower oil beforehand helps immensely with this. Place cloves for eyes, pumpkin seeds for ears and string for tails. Arrange the mice on a sheet of greaseproof paper and leave in a warm, dry place to harden for 24 hours.

USE When windy, eat 1–2 mice per day, remembering to remove the cloves first.

STORAGE Will keep in an airtight tin for up to 6 weeks.

IMMUNE SYSTEM

These remedies provide many of the vitamins and minerals you need to help build up your body's defences against infection and disease.

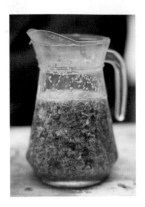

Nettle and Chamomile Tea for Hay Fever

Nettles contain chemicals with antihistamine and anti-inflammatory properties, which are thought to go some way towards depressing the immune system's allergic response. Locally produced honey is believed to give those suffering from flower pollen allergy some immunity from local pollens. Give this tea a go – it may help ease you through the annual hay fever season.

2–3 tbsp fresh nettles, or 1–2 tbsp dried

4 tsp fresh German chamomile (*Matricaria recutita*) or 2 tsp dried

1 tsp locally produced honey, to taste

1 Wash the fresh nettles well, then chop roughly with a large knife. Put the nettles, stalks and all, and chamomile into a glass teapot. Pour boiling water over and leave to steep for 5 minutes – this will also take the sting out of the nettles.

2 Strain into a tea cup and serve, adding 1 teaspoon of local honey, or to taste. This makes a pot equivalent to 3 cups.

USE Drink 3 cups a day while suffering from hay fever, for as long as you need it.

STORAGE Make fresh as you need it.

VARIATION ELDERFLOWER AND EYEBRIGHT TEA

Here's another potential weapon in the annual war against hay fever. Combine 100g dried elderflowers, 150g dried eyebright and 50g dried nettles (or use goldenrod). Use 1–2 teaspoons per cup of boiling water. Cover and leave to infuse for 10 minutes before straining, then drink. Take a cup as often as you wish.

To help ward off hay fever, start drinking plain elderflower tea (by infusing dried elderflowers, 1–2 tsp per cup of boiling water) at least 2–3 months before you normally start getting symptoms. Then when the hay fever season arrives, drink Elderflower and Eyebright Tea as needed.

'I'm not sure whether it's the weather or if it's psychosomatic, or what, but there seems to have been an effect from the tea, in terms of I'm not as bunged up as I used to be. I wouldn't say it's unblocked my nose but it's certainly stopped the itching in the back of my palate.' *Mike*

'When I tried the tea, about half an hour afterwards my eyes stopped streaming, my nose stopped running and my throat was soothed.' *Tracy*

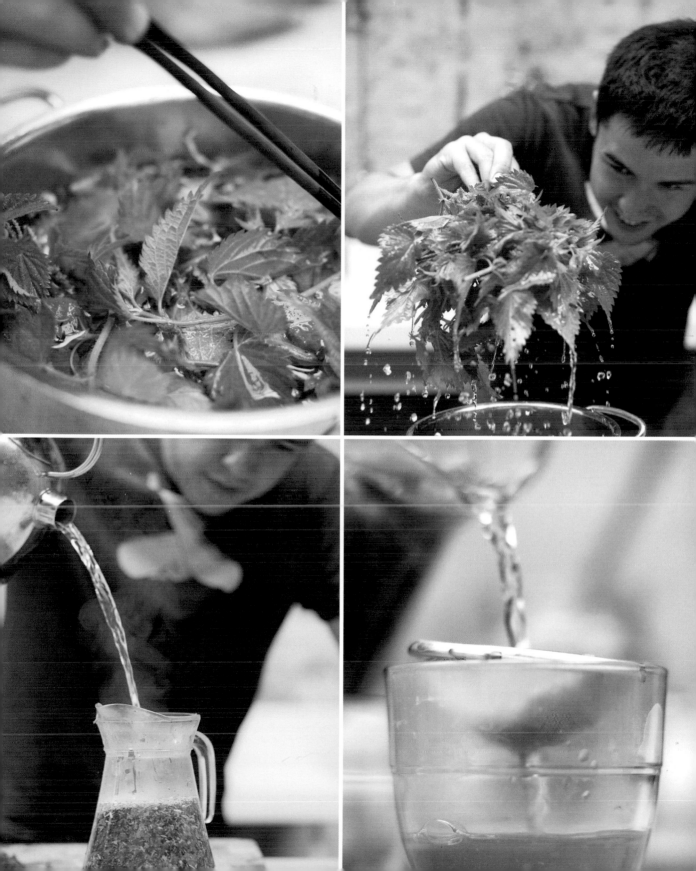

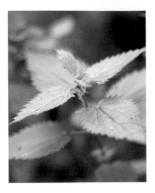

Restorative Nettle Tonic

Don't worry about not weeding your garden – the nettles will come in handy for this rich, restorative tonic. Nettles are highly nutritious, full of vitamins, minerals and chlorophyll, and the apricots contain iron to give your system a healthy winter boost. If you're trying to avoid yeast, use equal parts of vodka and water instead of the wine.

about 150g fresh nettles (pick fresh young growth)

about 400g apricots, fresh or dried and stoned

2 oranges (the more bitter, the better)

½ bottle red wine (or equal parts vodka and water), to cover

1 Fill half of a glass jar with rinsed, chopped nettles. Fill the other half with chopped apricots.

2 Peel the zest from the oranges and add to the mix. Cover with red wine. Leave for 2 weeks.

3 Strain the mixture through a sieve or wring it through a clean cloth into a large glass bowl. Press hard – the idea is to extract as much liquid as you possibly can. Then decant into sterilized glass bottles.

USE Take 2 teaspoons once or twice a day when you're feeling run down.

CAUTION Contains alcohol.

STORAGE Will keep for 6 months in the refrigerator.

gifting This tonic makes a great winter gift for anyone who's been ill or under the weather. Buy some lovely dark glass bottles new or second hand – or recycle ones you already have in your cupboard. Simply add a decorative, handwritten label. You can design a stick-on one, or cut a rectangle from a piece of card, punch a hole in a corner, then tie a pretty ribbon through, and hang round the neck of the bottle.

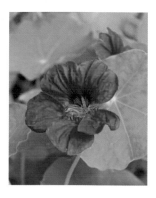

Four Flower Salad

In Britain, we grow flowers because they look good, but in other cultures they are thought of as a living supermarket cum pharmacy – prized for their culinary and medicinal properties. The simplest way to take in the goodness of flowers and herbs is to eat them raw, and this zingy mix contains anti-microbials and anti-inflammatories.
Use pot marigold (*Calendula officinalis*), not African or French marigold (*Tagetes*).

6 nasturtium
  flowerheads

6 marigold flowerheads

6 mallow flowers
  (common or marsh)

6 rocket flowerheads,
  nice and peppery

1 Wash the flowers and cut off any stalks or tough outer sepals. Sprinkle over a base of salad leaves. Dress the salad, and eat at once.

james's tip Fresh herbs can also be added to a green salad; the trick is not to use too much of one herb at a time, as it can drown the flavour of everything else. Try lemon balm leaves, mint, feathery fennel leaves, sage and thyme. Dandelion leaves are also good, but pick these when young, mainly in spring, because they become too bitter when they're old. Shred the leaves finely and try using a tablespoon of several varieties at a time.

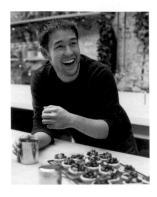

Roasted Cranberry Mince Pies

Instead of mincemeat in your mince pies this Christmas, try this healthy, roasted cranberry filling. The vitamin-packed cranberries taste sharp and tangy, and if eaten daily for a few weeks may even help prevent and ease the symptoms of cystitis. Makes about 15 pies.

Ikg cranberries, fresh or frozen

1 Bramley apple, chopped

1 tsp mixed spice

100g unsalted butter

100ml maple syrup

300g soft brown sugar

3 tbsp dark rum or Cointreau

100g candied orange peel

flour, for dusting

2 rolls ready-made shortcrust pastry

icing sugar, to dredge

1 Preheat the oven to 180°C (350°F).

2 Distribute the cranberries and chopped apple between two roasting tins. Sprinkle over the mixed spice and fleck with the butter. Drizzle the maple syrup over. Roast in the oven for 25–30 minutes, or until the fruit is slightly shrunken with a golden tan. If using frozen, you might need to roast for longer until the juices disappear.

3 Remove the roasted cranberries from the oven and place in a bowl. Mix in the sugar, rum or Cointreau and candied orange peel.

4 Sprinkle flour onto a work surface and roll out the pastry to a thickness of about 3mm. Using a 7cm cookie-cutter, cut out discs of pastry and place into a greased mince pie tin. Prick the base of each pie with a fork and bake in the oven for 15 minutes.

5 Remove from the oven, and spoon the cranberry filling into each pastry cup. Return to the oven to cook for another 5 minutes.

6 Leave the pies to cool, then dredge with icing sugar.

USE Eat 1 or 2 a day.

STORAGE Store in an airtight container and eat within 1 week.

gifting A jar of roasted cranberry filling makes a lovely homemade gift for anyone who enjoys cooking and who wants to make their own healthy mince pies at Christmas. Add a label with the storage details – the mixture will last for up to 1 month if kept in the refrigerator.

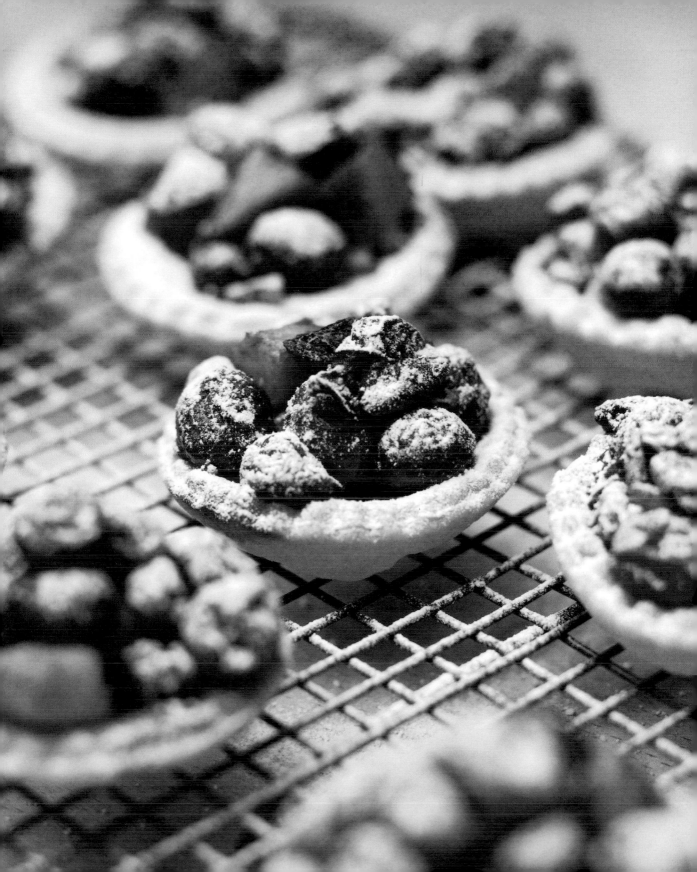

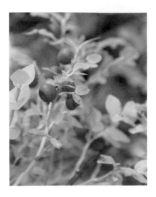

Simple Bilberry Tonic

Bilberries, also known as whortleberries (*Vaccinium myrtillus*), are a good source of vitamin C, antioxidants and anti-inflammatory free-radical scavengers called anthocyanosides. Harvest the berries from the heaths and moors in early August, then make up a big batch of this fruity general tonic to see you through the year. It can also help with eye disorders arising from diabetes and high blood pressure. If you can't get hold of bilberries, why don't you try making the tonic with blueberries?

500g bilberries (or as many as you can get), fresh or dried
water, to cover
sugar – 100g per 100ml bilberry liquid
vodka, brandy or whisky – 15ml per 100ml syrup

1 Put the bilberries in a pan and cover with cold water. Simmer until the bilberries are soft. Then press through a strainer or sieve with a wooden spoon to collect the pulp, discarding the seeds.

2 Measure the liquid/pulp and then return to the pan, adding sugar in the ratio of 100g sugar per 100ml bilberry liquid. Bring slowly to the boil, stirring occasionally, then simmer until thickened, usually about 30 minutes.

3 Allow to cool slightly, measure the syrup and add 15ml alcohol per 100ml syrup to act as a preservative. Bottle in small bottles (it must be used within 2 weeks after opening).

USE Take 1 teaspoon 3 times daily.

CAUTION Contains alcohol.

STORAGE Will keep for 1 year before opening. Keep in the refrigerator once opened, and use within 2 weeks.

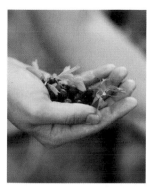

Three Fruits Vinegar for Colds and Flu

In late summer to early autumn, elderberries, hawthorn berries (haws) and rosehips ripen in the hedgerows at around the same time. Elderberry is a very useful antiviral and all three have high vitamin C content. Take this tonic vinegar to help build up your infection-fighting abilities during the long winter months.

100g hawthorn berries

100g elderberries

100g rosehips

cider vinegar, to cover

1 Place equal parts of hawthorn berries, elderberries and rosehips into a large, wide-mouthed jar. (Do not use jars with metal lids because these will corrode.) Cover generously with cider vinegar and allow to macerate for 10–14 days. Strain, label and bottle.

USE In the cold and flu season, take 1–2 tablespoons diluted in warm, boiled water in the morning before food.

STORAGE Will keep from 6 months to 1 year.

gifting Home-made herbal vinegars make practical gifts – they can be used in cooking as well as taken as a health tonic. Pour into a good-quality bottle, then seal. Make an ornamental label (with expiry date written on), and stick or string it round the bottle.

Port Winter Tonic

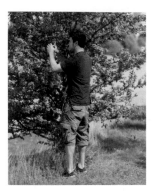

The unusual combination of ingredients in this tonic will give your immune system a timely winter boost. Hawthorn berries can help increase blood flow to the heart; lime flowers are gently relaxing; cinnamon and ginger help improve circulation; while goji berries are highly nutritious and help raise immunity. Try it as an alternative to mulled wine!

50g hawthorn berries, fresh or dried

50g goji berries, fresh or dried

3–4 tbsp lime (linden) flowers (*Tilia* spp.)

20g dried marshmallow root or 40g fresh mallow flowers

4 cinnamon sticks, broken up

5cm fresh ginger root, grated

1 litre port

Place all the plants in a large jar. Pour the port over, making sure to cover all the plant matter. Leave to macerate for 10–14 days. Strain and bottle.

USE Take 25–50ml on a winter evening.

CAUTION Contains alcohol.

STORAGE Will keep for up to 2 years.

gifting This tonic makes a great winter gift for anyone who's been ill or under the weather. Buy some lovely bottles new or second-hand – or recycle ones you already have in your cupboard. Tie or stick on a handwritten label, with the date and dosage clearly marked.

RESPIRATORY

Recipes to help minimize the symptoms of colds, coughs, sore throats, flu and other infections of the respiratory tract.

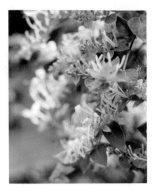

Honeysuckle and Jasmine Jelly for Sore Throats

In China, they often use medicinal jellies such as the renowned Gui Lin Gao (turtle essence jelly) instead of herbal teas. This is my take on Gui Lin Gao – though, thankfully, without the turtle! Honeysuckle is traditionally used in China as an anti-inflammatory and antiseptic, helpful with sore throats and respiratory complaints, and this soothing, delicately floral-scented jelly slips down a treat.

40g fresh honeysuckle (*Lonicera japonica*) flowers or 20g if using dried

10g fresh jasmine (*Jasminum grandiflorum*) flowers or 5g if using dried

500ml water

1 tsp green tea leaves

1 sachet powdered gelatine

4 tbsp orange blossom honey, or to taste

juice ½ lime

1 Wash the honeysuckle and jasmine flowers. Heat the water until hot (about the temperature of a hot bath), but do not allow it to boil. Pour into a jug with the tea leaves and flowers. Cover and leave to stand. Once cooled, place in the refrigerator for 24 hours.

2 Next day, strain the liquid into a pan, discarding the tea leaves and flowers. Heat the liquid gently until just below boiling point. Take off the heat, whisk in the gelatine, honey and lime juice. Pour into small tumblers or bowls, then cool and refrigerate until set like a loose jelly. This makes enough for 3 doses across 1 day.

3 Serve in tumblers or small bowls with jasmine and honeysuckle flowers for decoration.

USE Eat the jelly 2–3 times a day, or as required.

STORAGE Refrigerate and use within 2 days.

'It had a cooling, soothing effect when I was actually eating the jelly; the only thing I maybe don't like about this remedy is the fact that you can't take it out and about with you during the day; if it was something I could keep in my handbag it might be a little bit easier to have if a sore throat came on. The honeysuckle and jasmine did start to take effect and brought down the inflammation and helped cure the sore throat.' Jackie

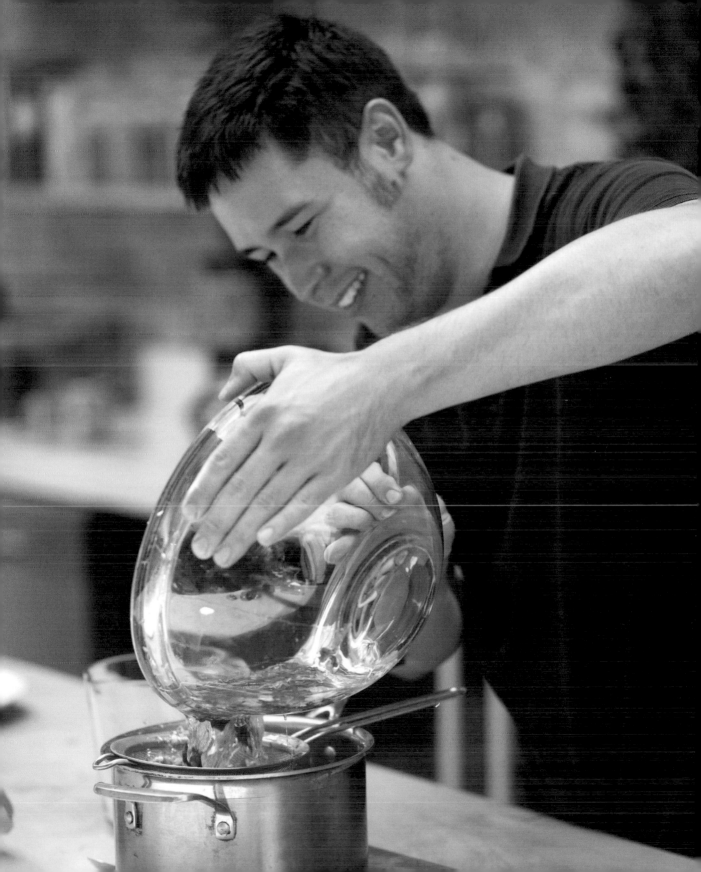

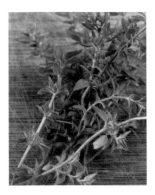

Thyme and Garlic Chest Rub

Thyme is an antiseptic and expectorant and garlic has antibiotic properties, helping to combat catarrh and soothe inflamed bronchial passages. Together they make a good (if whiffy!) rub for chesty colds, flu and sore throats – perhaps best used at night!

For the infused oil:

4–5 bulbs garlic

75g fresh or
   dried thyme

300–400ml olive oil,
   to cover

For the ointment:

300ml infused oil

25g beeswax

1 Peel the garlic cloves, and chop roughly. Layer the garlic and thyme in a clean jam jar until three-quarters full. Pour over the olive oil to the top of the jar, and seal. Place near a radiator for 10–14 days, giving the jar a shake and turn each day to let the warmth reach through.

2 Strain the oil through muslin or a jelly bag. Store in a clean jar in a cool, dark place. The infused oil can be rubbed into the chest, and will last for up to a year.

3 To make the ointment, put 300ml infused oil and the beeswax, chopped into small pieces, into a glass heatproof bowl, and stand over a saucepan of water. Bring the water to the boil, and simmer until the beeswax has melted, stirring occasionally. Remove the bowl from the hot water, cool for a short time, then pour into clean jars before it starts to set. Put the lid(s) on once the ointment has set.

USE Rub the oil or ointment on to the chest area as needed, especially before bed. The rub has a strong aroma, so wear an old T-shirt under your nightwear/pyjamas when you use it.

STORAGE Will keep for up to 1 year.

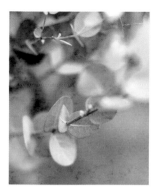

Elderflower and Eucalyptus Decongestant Throat Lozenges

Combining the goodness of elderflowers and elderberries and the decongestant properties of eucalyptus, these pleasant-tasting cough sweets contain antivirals and anti-inflammatories to help soothe sore throats and coughs. Carry a small tin around with you for use throughout the day. You'll find gum arabic in Asian food shops.

10–15 fresh elderflower heads

750ml freshly boiled water

2 tbsp linseed (flax seeds)

12 eucalyptus leaves

I cup gum arabic

3 tsp dried elderberries

250ml hot water

280g icing sugar

gifting Give a pretty tin of lozenges as a gift for someone feeling under the weather – pour the mixture into a baking tray, leave to cool a little, then score it into small squares with a sharp knife. Once cool, cut along the scores, roll the lozenges in icing sugar, put in the tin and then label.

1 Put the elderflower heads in a bowl and pour over the boiled water to make an infusion. Add the linseed and torn or bruised eucalyptus leaves, and leave for about 1 hour. It's ready when the pure watery liquid starts to have a similar consistency to egg white.

2 While the elderflower mixture is infusing, use a pestle and mortar to break up the gum arabic into the smallest pieces you can – this helps it to dissolve more easily. Add the dried elderberries to the mortar and crush.

3 Put the gum arabic mixture into a cup with the hot water. Stir until the granules of gum have turned into a thick, treacle-like consistency.

4 Strain the elderflower infusion, measure out 375ml and put into a pan. Add the gum arabic mixture and icing sugar and stir; the sugar acts as a preservative and gives it body.

5 Place the pan on a low heat and stir continuously for about 30 minutes, or until the mixture forms a very thick, golden syrup-like consistency and starts to come away from the sides of the pan. You can test it by dropping a tiny amount from a spoon into a glass of cold water – it's ready when the drop of mixture holds together and doesn't disperse into the water.

6 Pour the mixture onto a baking tray lined with greaseproof paper and leave to set. When hard, bash it with a rolling pin to get lozenge-sized pieces. Roll the lozenges in icing sugar to stop them sticking together, then store in an airtight tin.

USE Suck on a lozenge as needed to soothe a sore throat.

STORAGE Will keep in an airtight tin for at least 1 year.

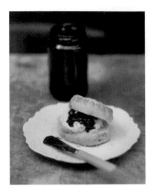

Eucalyptus and Elderberry Jelly

Elderberries are immunoprotective and inhibit viral replication – which means that when you're coming down with a cold or flu they can help to make symptoms shorter and less severe. Eat this delicious, health-promoting jelly on toast for breakfast, as an accompaniment to meats and cheese, or take a daily spoonful as you need it.

400g elderberries

1 Bramley apple

400ml water

juice of 1 lime

a few fresh
    eucalyptus leaves

whole dried chilli

500g granulated sugar

1 Wash the elderberries and apple. Chop the apple without peeling or coring. Put the elderberries, apple (including the core), water, lime juice, eucalyptus leaves and chilli into a pan and simmer for 15 minutes. Strain through a sieve, pressing with the back of a spoon to extract as much of the pulp as possible.

2 Place the elderberry liquid in a large pan and add the sugar. Bring to the boil, stirring occasionally to stop the sugar from burning, then simmer for another 30 minutes. If you have a jam thermometer to hand, the jelly reaches setting point at 105°C/221°F.

3 When it's ready, skim off any scum, then bottle in sterilized jam jars, putting a waxed disc, wax-side down, on top. Cover with a round of cellophane and secure with a rubber band or ribbon.

USE Take 1 generous tablespoon whenever you feel cold symptoms coming on.

STORAGE Will keep for up to 1 year in a cool, dark place. Once opened, store in the refrigerator.

gifting Little pots of Eucalyptus and Elderberry Jelly, decorated with cute cloth tops and a handwritten label tied on with ribbon, make great gifts for friends and neighbours.

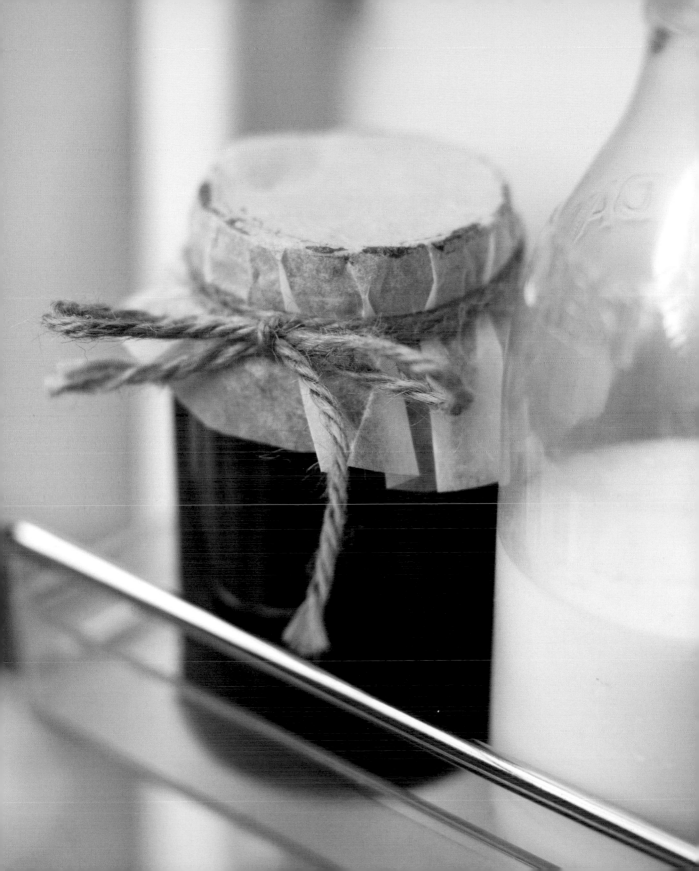

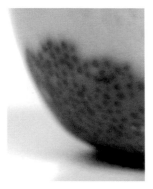

Elderberry Liqueur

This uses the same ingredients as the jelly on page 74, but in a medicinal hot toddy so you can have a quick shot when you're feeling under the weather with a cold or the flu. The chemicals found in elderberries help to stop viruses replicating and also boost the immune system, while eucalyptus and chilli help clear the nasal passages. Just pour a little in a glass and add hot water to dilute to your taste. If you use an eucalyptus-infused rum, so much the better (see Tip below).

250g Bramley apple

400g fresh elderberries, or 250g dried

500g sugar

2 tsp dried chilli flakes

3 tbsp eucalyptus leaves

300ml water

juice of 1 lime

100ml dark rum

1 Roughly chop the whole apple, skin, core and all. Pop in a pan and add all the remaining ingredients except the rum.

2 Simmer gently for 5 minutes, then take off the heat and strain through a fine sieve, pushing with the back of a spoon to extract as much pulp as possible.

3 Stir in the rum and bottle up.

USE For adults, take a little in a glass straight or dilute with hot water and drink as a hot toddy.

CAUTION Contains alcohol. Consideration should be taken when driving.

STORAGE Will keep for 1 year in a cool, dark place.

> **james's tip** To make an aromatic eucalyptus-infused rum, fill a glass jar with mature fresh eucalyptus leaves (the long, sickle-shaped ones) and cover with dark rum (40% alcohol, 80% proof), making sure that all the plant matter is submerged. Leave in a cool, dark place for a couple of weeks, then strain and use in the recipe above.

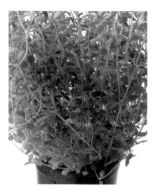

Thyme and Aniseed Cough Drops

These easy-to-make cough sweets are antiseptic, analgesic and very soothing. Thyme contains a powerful antimicrobial oil and is also slightly numbing, so very effective on sore throats.

6–8 tbsp chopped fresh thyme leaves

4 tsp aniseeds (*Pimpinella anisum*)

400ml cold water

400g sugar (white or brown)

icing sugar, for rolling

1 Put the thyme and aniseeds into a saucepan and cover with the water. Bring to the boil, then take off the heat and leave to infuse for 15 minutes.

2 Strain and add the white or brown sugar. Bring back to the boil, stirring occasionally, then boil until the mix is thick enough to leave a thread coming off the spoon. Be careful because the mixture is very hot and can give a nasty burn.

3 Drop teaspoonfuls of the mixture into a pan of cold water to form the cough drops. Take out immediately and leave to dry on a clean tea towel. Roll in icing sugar and store in a sealed container.

USE Suck on a cough drop as needed.

STORAGE Will keep in a sealed container for up to 2 years.

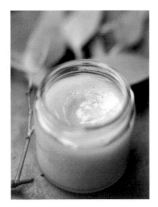

Eucalyptus Decongestant Rub for Sinusitis

If you've got a eucalyptus tree growing near you, it would be simply criminal not to use it. When extracted from the fresh leaves, eucalyptus oil smells rich, buttery and sweet – much more appealing than the commercially prepared essential oil, which smells a bit clinical and chemically to me. Use this rub as a fragrant natural decongestant and expectorant for blocked sinuses and head colds.

100g mature
  eucalyptus leaves

10g ginger

¼ tsp ground
  black pepper

200g white
  petroleum jelly

20 drops peppermint
  essential oil

1 Chop the eucalyptus leaves and ginger and place in a glass heatproof bowl. Add the ground pepper and petroleum jelly and mix everything together with your fingers.

2 Place the glass bowl, covered, over a pan of boiling water to make a double boiler. Leave to heat for 1 hour, making sure the water does not boil dry.

3 Take off the heat and strain the mixture. Stir in the peppermint oil and bottle in a wide-mouthed jar.

USE Once a day, rub well into the chest and throat area. The rub can help you get a good night's sleep if applied before bed.

CAUTION Do not use on broken skin. If any reddening or irritation occurs, wash off immediately.

STORAGE Will keep for up to 1 year.

VARIATION EUCALYPTUS INHALATION

A eucalyptus inhalation can help soothe a congested respiratory tract. Take a handful of eucalyptus leaves, break or chop them, place in a wide bowl and pour freshly boiled water over. Alternatively, you can put 1 teaspoon of the Eucalyptus Rub into a bowl of boiling water. Stir and allow to cool slightly. Then lean over the bowl – being careful to remain at least 30cm above the hot water – and wrap a towel around your head and over the bowl. Inhale the vapours for a few minutes, once a day as needed.

james's tip When making recipes with eucalyptus, always choose the mature leaves – they're long and sickle-shaped – not the round, juvenile leaves. The older leaves contain a higher concentration of the oil and active ingredients.

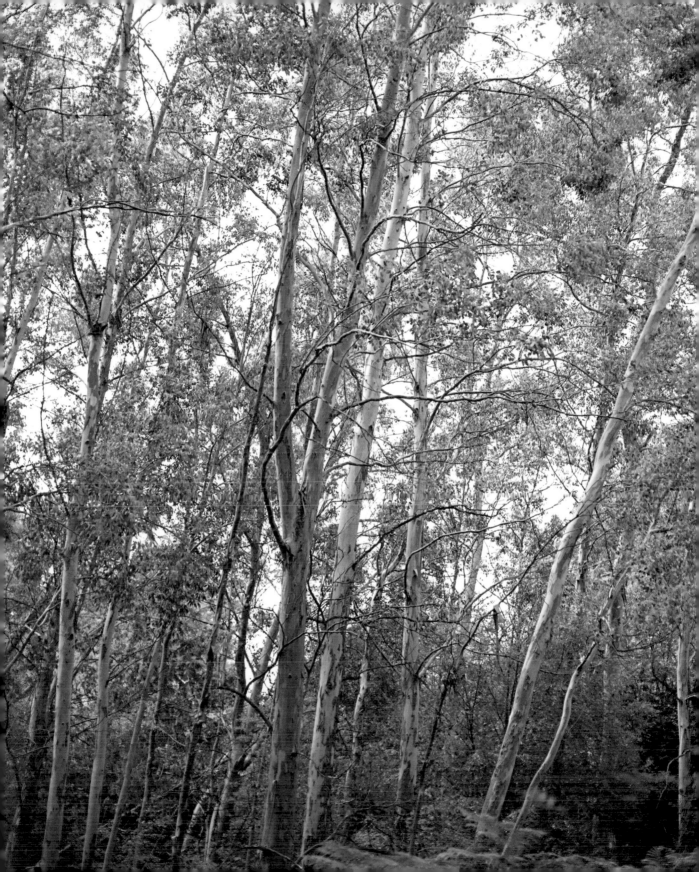

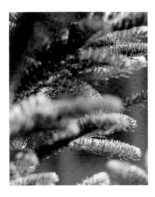

Fir Tree and Calamondin Hot Toddy

Try this soothing and aromatic hot toddy to help ease the symptoms of colds and flu. Use the freshest fir needles you can find – trimmings from your new Christmas tree, for example – as they contain greater concentrations of the essential plant compounds. Use fir needles from the Fraser fir *(Abies fraseri)*, or Norway spruce *(Picea abies)*.

For the echinacea-infused rum:

15g fresh echinacea root (or 10g if using dried)

100ml white rum

For the hot toddy:

120ml fir needles

1 star anise

3 calamondin oranges or 1 lime, sliced

2 tbsp eucalyptus honey

pinch of black pepper

250ml boiling water

1 shot (28ml) echinacea-infused rum (see above)

1 tsp unsalted butter

1 To make the echinacea-infused rum, combine the echinacea root and rum and leave to steep in a cool, dark place for 2 weeks. Strain out the echinacea and bottle up. The mixture will keep in a cool, dark place for up to 1 year.

2 To make the hot toddy, strip the needles from the fir branches until you have 120ml.

3 Put the needles in a teapot or bowl with the star anise and halved sliced calamondin oranges or lime, honey and black pepper, and pour over the freshly boiled water. Cover and leave to steep for 15 minutes.

4 Strain into a pan, and reheat on the stove.

5 Once reheated, add the echinacea-infused rum and butter until melted. Stir, then serve in a large cup.

USE For adults, drink 1 cup only in the evening or before bedtime.

CAUTION Contains alcohol. Consideration should be made when driving.

STORAGE Best made fresh for use at once.

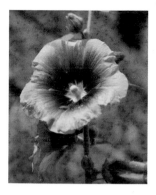

Hollyhock Cough Syrup

Hollyhock flowers soothe irritated mucous membranes and can help ease a dry cough. They bloom prolifically in July and August – choose dark-coloured flowers to make a beautiful jewel-like syrup (although light-coloured flowers work just as well!).

about 20 heaped tbsp hollyhock flowers, depending on the size of your jar

400g white sugar, approx

brandy – 15ml per 100ml syrup

1 Lightly bruise the hollyhock flowers.

2 In a wide-mouthed jar, layer the flowers to a height of 3cm, then top with a layer of sugar, also 3cm high. Continue until the jar is full, alternating flowers and sugar, and ending with a sugar layer.

3 Leave in a warm place until most of the sugar is dissolved. This can take up to 1 month.

4 Strain off the flowers and throw away any undissolved sugar. (Alternatively, use it in cooking – to poach fruit, for example.)

5 Measure the syrup, and add 15ml of brandy per 100ml syrup to preserve. Stir well. Pour into a sterilized dark glass bottle.

USE Take 2 tablespoons as required, to sooth a dry cough.

STORAGE Keep refrigerated and use within 2 weeks once opened.

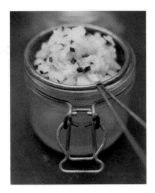

Onion Gargle for Throat Infections

Packed with antibiotics, antioxidants and anti-inflammatories, this fiery onion and chilli gargle will help fight infection and soothe the irritation and discomfort of a sore throat.

I onion

½ fresh red chilli

juice of 2 lemons

I tsp salt

sprig of parsley

1 Chop the onion and chilli finely and place in a bowl. Add the lemon juice and salt. Leave to stand for 1 hour in the refrigerator.

2 Strain and use as a gargle. After gargling, chew on a sprig of parsley to freshen breath.

USE Gargle daily, as soon as you feel a sore throat coming on, then spit out rather than swallow.

STORAGE Best made and used fresh each day.

'It's obviously not delightful, but it's alright! It did help, it took the edge off things, but it did wear off throughout the day.' Louise

'This remedy I'll definitely use again. I gargled twice, once in the evening and once in the afternoon, and by the next day my scratchiness had gone and I could breathe better.' Jade

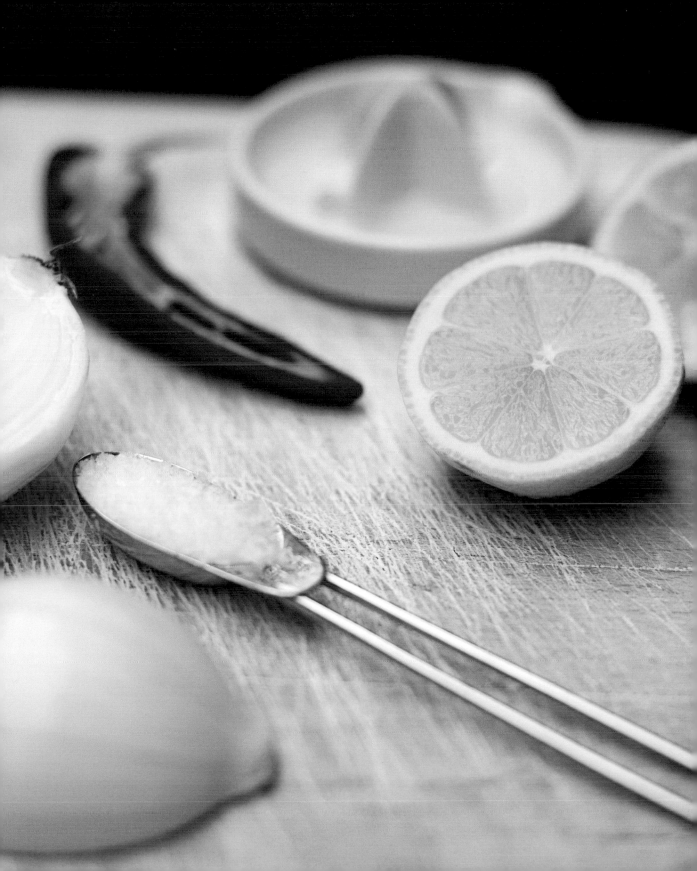

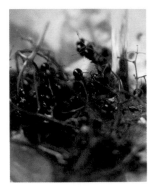

Elderberry and Ginger Cold and Flu Tonic

Thousands of years ago, Hippocrates and Pliny were writing about the health-giving properties of the elder tree. Its beautiful black berries – which fruit prolifically in late summer/early autumn – are anti-viral and have been shown to help minimize and soothe cold and flu symptoms. This tonic has an extra zap and flavour from the ginger. Take as soon as you feel a cold coming on.

3–4 tbsp cinnamon quills or sticks, broken up

30g fresh ginger root, roughly sliced

10–12 tbsp elderberries, fresh or dried

1.7 litre water

1 tbsp meadowsweet flowers

honey, lemon or brandy, to taste

1 Put the cinnamon, ginger, elderberries and water in a large stainless steel pan and bring to the boil. Simmer for 30 minutes.

2 Turn off the heat, then add the meadowsweet flowers and leave to infuse for 10 minutes. Strain into a large bowl. Add honey, lemon or brandy to taste. Pour into a thermos.

USE Adults: best drunk the same day, freely at the onset of cold/flu symptoms.

CAUTION Do not give to children under 16 due to the meadowsweet. Don't eat raw elderberries, though cooked ones are fine! If pregnant or allergic to aspirin, leave out the meadowsweet.

STORAGE Will keep in the refrigerator for up to 36 hours.

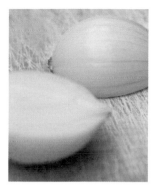

Onion Syrup

This syrup is traditionally used to help clear phlegm from the respiratory tract. You can make it with garlic instead of onion, and it will be just as effective (although a little smellier!).

about 2 large onions, depending on jar size

about 400g sugar (any kind will do)

1 Roughly chop the onions, and place a layer in a clean jar (an old sterilized jam jar is fine). Cover with a layer of sugar, then continue to layer onion and sugar until the jar is full – you might need more or less onion and sugar, depending on the size of your jar. Seal the jar.

2 Leave for a few hours or overnight to allow the sugar to draw the liquid out of the onions, producing a syrup – at this stage, it's fun for children to watch the syrup appearing in the jar.

3 Next day, if there is still a lot of sugar at the bottom of the jar, add some more onion. Or if the onion bits are still fairly large (they will shrink as the moisture is drawn out), add more sugar.

4 As soon as there is any liquid, you can start taking the syrup. After about 1 day, strain all the onion bits out, and store the syrup in the refrigerator.

USE Adults and teenagers: take 4 teaspoons in the morning and early afternoon. Children over 2: take 2 teaspoons morning and early afternoon. Avoid taking before bedtime (coughing up phlegm during the night will disturb sleep).

STORAGE Will keep for several days in the refrigerator.

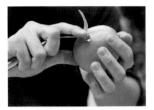

Cold and Flu Chai

Drink this warming, aromatic chai to help relieve the symptoms of a feverish cold or flu.

5cm fresh ginger, grated

1–3 cinnamon sticks

small pinch of black peppercorns, crushed

small pinch of whole cloves

6 cardamom pods

peel of 1 orange

600ml water

1 tbsp yarrow flowers

1 tbsp meadowsweet flowers

300ml milk

honey, to taste

1 Place the ginger, cinnamon (broken up), peppercorns, cloves, cardamom (broken open) and orange peel into a pan with the water. Bring to the boil and reduce by half to about 300ml; this will take about 15 minutes at a rolling boil.

2 Add the yarrow and meadowsweet flowers and the milk and allow to heat through. Strain, and sweeten with honey if required.

USE This makes enough for 2–3 cups. Pour it into a thermos and drink hot throughout the day, being sure to have a cup before going to bed at night.

CAUTION Not to be given to children under 16, due to the meadowsweet. If pregnant or allergic to aspirin, leave out the meadowsweet.

STORAGE Will keep for 1–2 days in the refrigerator, but best made fresh at the beginning of each day.

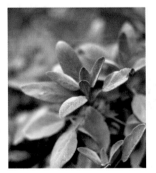

Sage and Marigold Gargle for Sore Throats

Gargles can provide instant relief from sore, irritated throats, and this one packs a big herbal punch. Sage and marigold are both antiseptic and antimicrobial; echinacea slows infection and can boost the immune system; cloves are also antiseptic and – as any dentist will tell you – act as a local anaesthetic.

50g echinacea root

20g sage

20g marigold flowers (*Calendula officinalis*)

½ tsp cloves

200ml vodka

1 Put all the herbs into the vodka and seal in a jar. Leave in a warm place for 10–14 days, shaking every day. Strain, then bottle.

USE Take 1 tablespoon diluted in a small glass of warm, boiled water. Gargle and swallow (or spit if you don't like the taste!). Repeat throughout the day as needed.

CAUTION Contains alcohol.

STORAGE Will keep for up to 2 years.

MUSCULAR
AND JOINTS

Easy-to-make plant remedies that help soothe the pain and inflammation associated with aching muscles, stiff joints and chronic conditions such as rheumatism and arthritis.

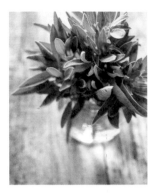

Vinegar Compress for Swollen Joints

Vinegar can help bring out bruises and reduce painful joint swelling. Combined with anti-inflammatory and healing plants such as sage and yarrow, it makes a soothing hot or cold compress for sprains, bruises and joints.

3–4 tbsp sage leaves, fresh

3–4 tbsp yarrow

3–4 tbsp plantain leaves

500ml malt vinegar approx, to cover

Roughly chop the sage, yarrow and plantain leaves and place in a wide-mouthed jar. Cover with the malt vinegar. Put the bottle in a warm place for 10–14 days. Then strain and bottle.

USE Heat a muslin cloth in hot water (as hot as is bearable), squeeze out the water, splash some of the vinegar on to the cloth and apply to sprains, strains and bruises. Repeat a couple of times, changing the compress as it cools.

USE Apply a compress 2–3 times a day until the bruise or swelling has gone.

STORAGE Will keep for up to 1 year.

VARIATION COOLING COMPRESS

As a cooling compress for hot, swollen joints or hot tension headaches, keep the infused vinegar in the refrigerator. Splash the cold vinegar on to a muslin cloth and apply to the affected area. Refresh as the compress warms up.

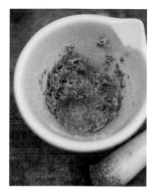

Turmeric 'Teh Halia' for Arthritis and Psoriasis

My version of Teh Halia – a Malay chai-type drink literally meaning 'ginger tea' – contains turmeric, traditionally used as an anti-inflammatory, antioxidant and mild anaesthetic to help soothe sore, stiff, arthritic joints and other inflammatory conditions such as psoriasis and Crohn's disease. The ginger (best used fresh) and black pepper both help the body absorb the curcumin, the active ingredient in turmeric. This makes enough for one frothy, golden cup of Teh.

3 sticks fresh turmeric or 4g dried

thumb-sized piece fresh ginger root

few pinches black pepper

250ml whole milk

250ml water

I tsp black tea leaves

palm sugar, to taste (or maple syrup or brown sugar)

1 Peel and chop the fresh turmeric, if using (being careful not to stain surfaces or hands). Peel and grate the ginger. Put into a mortar (with the dried turmeric, if using) and add a few pinches of black pepper, then pound with the pestle until you get a smooth paste.

2 Combine the paste with the milk, water and tea leaves in a pan and simmer on a low heat for 10 20 minutes, or until the liquid is reduced by half. Strain. Sweeten with palm sugar to taste, and stir.

3 Before drinking, pour the Teh between two containers, holding them the maximum width apart to aerate the tea as much as possible and produce a froth on top. Despite not having too much of a medicinal effect on the remedy, this is more than just a flamboyant whim. Aerating the mix improves its flavour by making it easier for your tongue to perceive the chemicals that give the drink its unique taste.

USE Make the Teh up as you need it, and drink at once. Take daily to help with arthritis, aches and pains in the joints, psoriasis, Crohn's disease and other inflammatory conditions.

STORAGE The paste keeps for up to 1 month in the refrigerator.

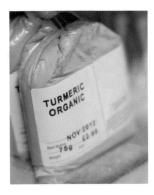

Quick-Fix Teh Halia

This is an instant, dried version of the Teh Halia on page 89 that's much easier to use on a daily basis than making up fresh. This recipe gives you 2 weeks' worth of dried Teh. Just pop it into an airtight tin, and you can take it with you to make up and drink wherever you are.

112g dried turmeric

28g dried ginger

½ tsp black pepper

25g black tea leaves

140g brown granulated sugar

❚ Stir all the ingredients together, then store in a dry, airtight tin. Makes 14 cups – or one a day.

USE To make up into a Teh, place 5–6 teaspoons of the mixture in a pan with 250ml whole milk and 250ml water, then simmer over a low heat for 10–20 minutes, or until reduced by half. Strain and serve.

STORAGE The mixture will keep in an airtight tin for 2 weeks.

👍 james's tip Turmeric is traditionally used as a fabric dye throughout Asia, and the rich, fabulous orange colour is evidence of how packed it is with antioxidants since the same chemicals that give it its colour are those which have the medicinal benefit. But be warned: the fresh root will stain surfaces and hands just as effectively as it stains textiles! You can use dried turmeric instead if you prefer; it won't stain as badly and is just as medicinally effective (provided it hasn't been languishing on your spice shelves for years).

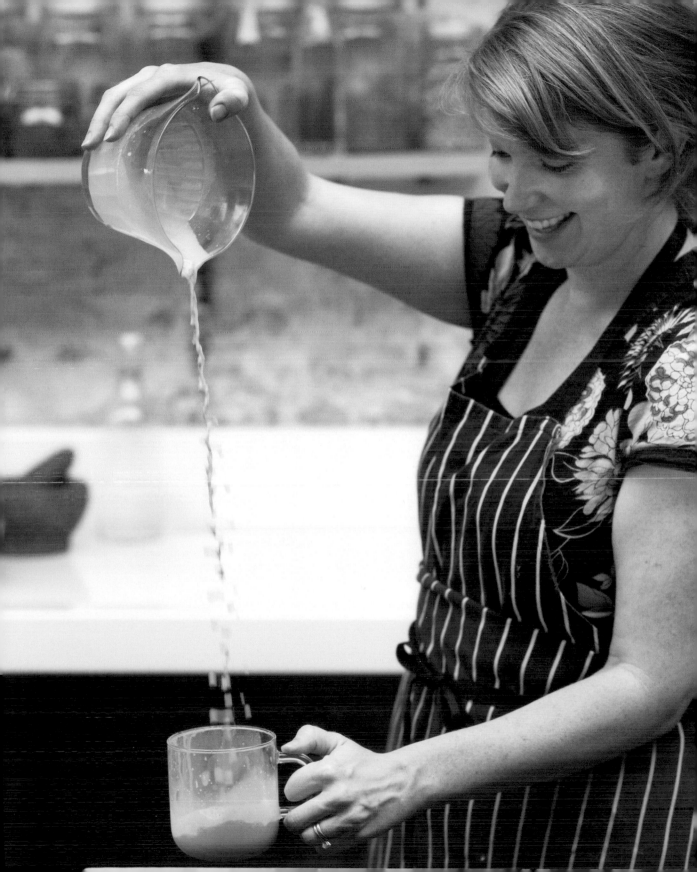

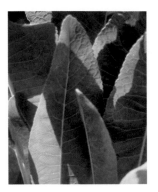

Horseradish and Mustard Balm for Arthritic Joints

A deep-heat treatment that can help invigorate circulation and increase blood flow to sore and swollen joints. The mustard has anaesthetic qualities, so it acts as a local pain reliever too.

3 whole roots (about 10cm long) fresh horseradish

200g white petroleum jelly

1½ tbsp black mustard seeds, bruised

½ tsp cayenne pepper powder

400ml vodka (or whisky, if you prefer)

1 Grate the horseradish. Take extra care because it makes the eyes stream even more than onions do! Place the horseradish and petroleum jelly in a saucepan and heat gently for 30 minutes. Strain through a coarse sieve while still warm.

2 In a separate saucepan, mix the bruised black mustard seeds and cayenne pepper with the vodka or whisky and heat gently for 10 minutes (do not boil).

3 Strain the warm vodka/whisky liquid into the petroleum and horseradish wax. Mix together well. Pour into wide-mouthed balm pots, and allow to cool before sealing.

USE Massage into aching joints before bed, then wrap with a cloth and leave on overnight. Wash off in the morning.

CAUTION Wash hands thoroughly after applying this preparation. Do not allow balm to come into contact with eyes, nose or mucus membranes.

STORAGE Will keep for up to 6 months.

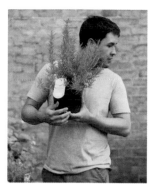

Rosemary and Clove Liniment for Rheumatic Relief

A liniment – more liquid than a cream – rubs in very easily over sore rheumatic joints and muscles. This one contains rosemary to help boost circulation, and cloves for their valuable pain-relieving effect.

3–4 tbsp fresh
   rosemary leaves,
   stripped
   from the woody stems

200ml sunflower oil,
   approx to cover

I tbsp whole cloves

100ml vodka (or whisky,
   if you prefer)

a pinch of borax powder
   (available from
   pharmacies)

1 Fill a jar with the rosemary leaves, then pour the sunflower oil over to cover. Seal and leave in a warm place to infuse for 2 weeks, or until the oil has taken on colour. Strain into a bottle.

2 Put the cloves and vodka (or whisky) in a pan and heat gently for about 5 minutes to release the oil from the cloves. Do not boil; if you can smell the cloves strongly, you are losing the volatile oils. Strain the tincture and allow to cool.

3 Put 100ml of the infused oil and 100ml of the clove tincture in a bottle. Add a pinch of borax powder, which acts as a weak emulsifier, and shake vigorously to mix. Seal.

USE Massage into affected areas as often as needed.

CAUTION Wash hands thoroughly after applying this preparation.

STORAGE Will keep for up to 1 year.

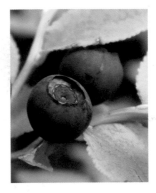

Bilberry and Marshmallow Munch for Aching Joints

Bilberries contain anthocyanosides, free-radical scavengers that have positive anti-inflammatory effects throughout the body. I think of this as a 'herbal glucosamine', which can help ease the joint stiffness and aches that often come with ageing. Munch on a little every day. Rosewater can be found at supermarkets and Asian food shops. Gotu kola can be bought from herbal suppliers, as *Centella asiatica*.

To make the rose and mallow syrup:

400g manuka honey

200ml rosewater (from supermarkets/ Asian food shops)

60g marshmallow root, dried

Powdered herbs:

80g bilberries, dried and powdered

80g rosehips, dried and powdered

55g gotu kola, dried and powdered

¼ whole nutmeg, grated

1 Mix together the manuka honey and rosewater in a sterilized, sealable jar, then add the marshmallow root. Steep for 2 weeks, shaking or stirring daily until it forms a syrup.

2 Strain and squeeze out the syrup through two layers of muslin.

3 Measure out 150ml syrup and mix in the powdered herbs. Mould into a ball or giant tablet and refrigerate in a sealed container.

USE Eat 1 generous teaspoon daily.

STORAGE Will keep in the refrigerator for up to 3 months.

 james's tip Any extra rose and mallow syrup can be taken internally as a gentle laxative; 1 dose is 2 teaspoons.

EMOTIONAL, HORMONAL AND HEADACHES

Whether you are feeling stressed, tired and overwrought, or suffering frequent headaches or migraine, or are just a bit under the weather, these remedies can give both sexes an emotional lift.

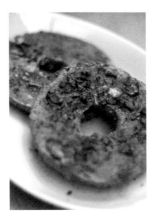

Herb Butter for Migraine Prevention

Eating a couple of feverfew leaves every day can help prevent migraine attacks and is definitely worth trying if you're prone to that kind of headache. Trouble is, they taste intensely bitter – so I've disguised the flavour here by loading up on the tarragon, lemon and parsley. The result is a rich herbal spread, which is my way of justifiably calling butter a health food. Fresh feverfew is not available over winter, but you can make and freeze enough of this herb butter to last you until next spring.

3 tsp fresh feverfew leaves (approx 20 leaves)

2 tsp fresh tarragon

2 tsp flat leaf parsley

I heaped tsp lemon zest

2 tsp powdered ginger

100g unsalted butter, at room temperature

salt and pepper to taste

1 On a wooden board, finely chop the feverfew leaves, tarragon and parsley. Add the lemon zest and ginger. Mix in the soft butter and salt and pepper to taste, and work until the herbs are evenly distributed throughout the butter.

2 Place the herb butter on a sheet of greaseproof paper and form into a long sausage shape. Mark lightly into seven equal portions (about 15g each), enough for a week's supply. Roll up the paper and seal at both ends.

USE Eat one 15g portion daily on bread or toast to prevent migraine.

CAUTION Do not use if you are pregnant or breastfeeding, under 18, or have a stomach or mouth ulcer. If on medication, check with your doctor or pharmacist before using. Discontinue if you feel nausea or other discomfort. As with other painkillers after long-term use, you might experience 'rebound' symptoms such as headaches when you stop. If so, consult your doctor or pharmacist.

STORAGE Will keep in the refrigerator for 1 week or in the freezer for up to 6 months.

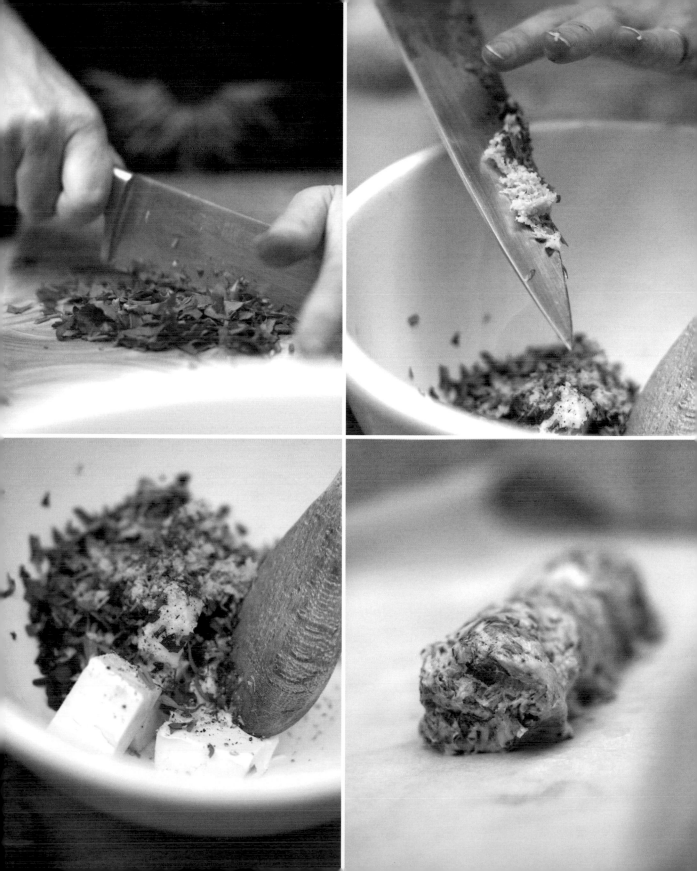

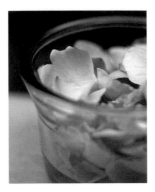

Rose and Chocolate Shot

This fabulous mood-enhancer combines two amazing flavours and colours. Rose is traditionally thought of as a heart tonic and anti-anxiety herb, and flavonoid-packed dark chocolate (not the sugary goo from confectioners) is good for heart health as well as acting as a mild stimulant and antidepressant. Don't be daunted by this recipe – both the tincture and syrup keep well, so you can make a batch and have a quick shot whenever your mood needs a lift. To make the rose syrup, any scented rose will do; Damasks and *Rosa gallica* are particularly good.

To make the chocolate tincture:

600g good-quality cocoa nibs (roasted cocoa beans)

vodka (80% proof or 40% alcohol), to cover

1 Using a pestle and mortar, crush 200g of the cocoa nibs to a coarse consistency. (Do not crush to a fine powder; the released fat content will make the mix gooey and unusable.)

2 Place the nibs in a jam jar and cover with vodka to about 1cm above the level of the cocoa nibs. Screw the lid on, set aside, and shake the jar daily for 5 days or more.

3 At this point, you will have a weak chocolate tincture. To make it stronger, strain the tincture you have made and put to one side, discarding the used cocoa nibs. Repeat Steps 1–2 twice more with the remaining cocoa nibs, using the strained alcohol mixture. Do this three times in total – it should take at minimum 15 days. After the final straining, pour the tincture into a dark jar and seal.

To make the rose syrup:

250g pink or red rosebuds or petals

250ml water

500g unrefined white sugar

1 Remove all stalks and green parts of the rose if using buds (this will remove tannins and create a better scent and taste). Rinse the roses under cold water. Pat dry.

2 Heat the water, preferably in a glass or ceramic pan, until it begins to boil and then reduce the heat. Add the roses to the water and cover. Leave to steep on a gentle heat for 20 minutes. Do not allow to boil. Strain through muslin into a jug or bowl.

3 Pour the strained infusion back into the original pan. Place the pan on a gentle heat and add the sugar. Stir with a wooden spoon until all the sugar is dissolved. Remove from the heat and leave to cool. Place in a sterilized bottle and seal.

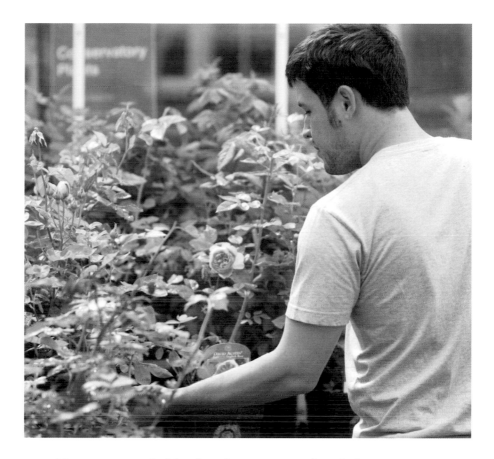

USE Measure out 10ml of the chocolate tincture and 20ml of rose syrup in a shot glass. Do not mix together – the layers of cocoa tincture and rose syrup should remain separate. Drink it down all in one, like a shot! To make the shot more warming, add a pinch of cayenne pepper to the cocoa nib tincture and stir before taking.

CAUTION Contains alcohol.

STORAGE The tincture will keep for up to 5 years in a dark jar. The syrup will keep for up to 1 year in a cool dark place.

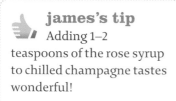

james's tip Adding 1–2 teaspoons of the rose syrup to chilled champagne tastes wonderful!

gifting Arrange two shot glasses, a packet of cocoa nibs and a quarter bottle of vodka in a pretty box, pad around with tissue paper, and slip a copy of the Rose and Chocolate Shot recipe inside. Cover with cellophane, tie a big bow round and you have a highly original gift.

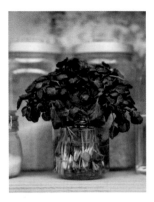

Restorative Watercress and Pear Soup

This vitamin- and mineral-rich soup is a delicious natural pick-me-up when you're anaemic or feeling tired and run down. People think spinach is rich in iron, but the dark green leaves of watercress contain significantly more iron as well as vitamin C, which helps your body absorb the iron more efficiently. The pears contain many vitamins and minerals, are a good source of soluble fibre, and add a note of sweetness to the taste; and the ginger, garlic and chilli give an extra, warming zing.

I large bunch
   spring onions

5 garlic cloves

I thumb-size piece
   of ginger

2 tbsp olive oil

2 small potatoes

750ml vegetable stock

2 pears

2 bunches watercress

salt and pepper, to taste

sprinkle of crushed chilli
   and extra slivers
   of pear (optional),
   to garnish

1 Chop the spring onions and garlic. Peel and finely grate the ginger (or use a garlic press) to extract the juice.

2 In a large sauté pan, heat the olive oil and gently fry the spring onions and garlic for 10 minutes. Slice the potatoes and add to the pan with the stock. Squeeze in the juice from the grated ginger, discarding the fibrous pulp. Simmer for 20 minutes.

3 Dice the pears. Wash and chop the watercress. Put the pears and watercress into a blender, add the potato stock mix, and purée.

4 Add salt and pepper to taste, and serve the soup garnished with pieces of pear and chilli and a dash of olive oil.

USE Good nutrition is all about balance, and I think of this soup as being a nutritional booster – it's a healthy move if you can incorporate it into your diet once or even twice a week. On other days, eat plenty of dark green leafy vegetables, beans, lentils, cereals and nuts, which are also good sources of iron.

STORAGE This makes about 3 bowls. Best eaten within 2 days.

> **james's tip** I don't bother to peel potatoes or pears in this or any other recipe – I always think it's healthier, albeit lazier, to leave the skin on. Though feel free if you prefer to peel …

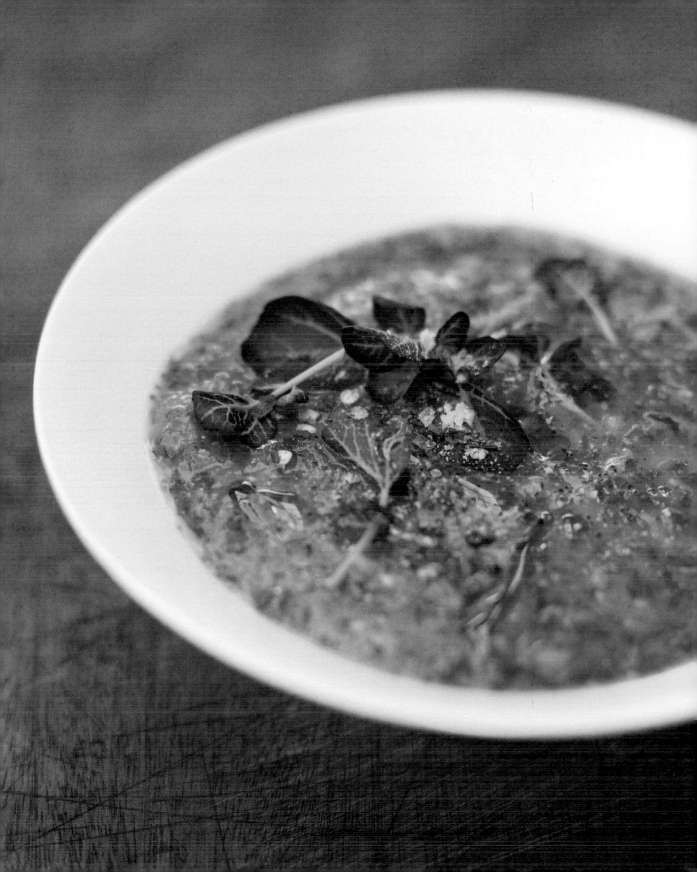

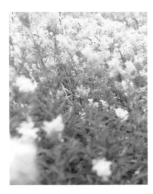

Meadowsweet Cordial

Sweet, fragrant and with the power to relieve pain – it is hard to see how a remedy could get any better. This flowery syrup is based on the frothy blossoms of meadowsweet plants, traditionally used to treat headaches and fevers, and one of the plants from which aspirin was first derived. The very word 'aspirin' comes from the plant's old Latin name, *Spiraea*. With a flavour like a fizzy cross between elderflower and marzipan, meadowsweet flowers can be found in damp meadows and along banks and ditches all over Britain.

1 lemon

10–20 meadowsweet
   flowerheads

180ml water

180g sugar

1 Grate the rind from the lemon and squeeze the juice. Place the lemon rind and juice with all the other ingredients in a stainless steel pan. Bring gently to the boil, stirring occasionally, then simmer for 10 minutes.

2 Strain into one or two small sterilized bottles and allow to cool before sealing. (It's best to make small amounts because the syrup can go mouldy within a week of opening.) For a year-round supply, simply pop a couple of plastic bottles of the cordial in the freezer, where they will last for at least one year.

USE Dilute with water for a refreshing drink.

CAUTION Should not be given to children under 16. Don't take if pregnant or allergic to aspirin.

STORAGE Keep in the refrigerator, and use within 1 week. Or in the freezer for up to 1 year.

james's tip For children aged 2–16, you can use other fragrant summer-flowering herbs such as lemon balm or elderflower instead of the meadowsweet. Just substitute 3–4 heaped tablespoons of the fresh flowers for the meadowsweet, and follow the recipe above.

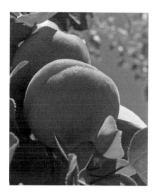

Meadowsweet and Peach Sorbet

Pairing the pain-relieving properties of meadowsweet with the flavour of fragrant summer peaches, this cooling, fruity sorbet is a true guiltless pleasure. For the meadowsweet cordial, see the recipe opposite.

3 ripe peaches

1 orange

120ml meadowsweet cordial

2 egg whites

1 Peel and stone the peaches and pop them into the blender.

2 Add the grated zest and juice of the orange, as well as the meadowsweet cordial, and whizz for a few seconds.

3 Put in a plastic container and leave in the freezer until just beginning to freeze (about 1 hour, depending on your freezer). Remove from the freezer and beat thoroughly.

4 Whip the egg whites until stiff, then fold into the peach mixture and freeze until ready to eat.

USE Gorge on as required.

CAUTION Should not be given to children under 16. Don't take if pregnant or allergic to aspirin.

STORAGE Will keep for up to 3 months in a sealed container in the freezer.

 james's tip For children aged 2–16, make the sorbet with lemon balm or elderflower cordial instead of the meadowsweet cordial.

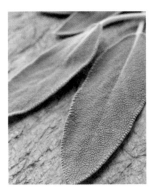

Sage Beer

A tasty general tonic if you're feeling run down and tired. Sage has long been considered a cure-all, and this brew also contains B vitamins, which support the nervous system. Find malt syrup from health food shops.

450g malt syrup

30g fresh sage leaves, plus an extra sprig

112g brown sugar

4.5 litres water

brewer's yeast (use the amount directed on the packet for 4.5 litres liquid)

a few teaspoons sugar

1 Boil the malt syrup, sage leaves, sugar and water together for 30 minutes in a stainless steel pot. Strain the liquid into a glass carboy. Once cooled to body temperature, add an extra sprig of fresh sage and the yeast. Fit an airlock and allow to ferment until done (about 2 weeks).

2 Pour into sterilized 330ml screw-top or swing-top bottles (you'll need about 6) with ½ teaspoon sugar per bottle – this is called 'priming' and helps get a nice fizz. Allow to ferment for at least another 2 weeks before drinking.

USE Drink a chilled 330ml bottle a day for 1–2 weeks.

CAUTION Contains alcohol. Home-made beers can be quite strong, so don't drive or use heavy machinery after drinking.

STORAGE Will keep for up to 1 year in the refrigerator. Once opened, the beer won't keep.

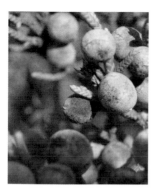

Soothing Rub for Period Pain

Rosemary and juniper join forces to improve circulation, with juniper also providing anti-inflammatory and pain-relieving properties. If you're not keen on the smell of rosemary, feel free to ditch it and use the infused juniper oil on its own.

For the infused oil:
100g juniper berries

about 250ml olive or
   almond oil, to cover

For the rub:
50ml infused juniper oil

20 drops rosemary
   essential oil

1 Place the juniper berries in a glass jar and pour over the olive or almond oil, then seal and leave for 2 weeks to infuse. Strain.

2 Place 50ml infused juniper oil in a small jar, add 20 drops rosemary essential oil and shake well.

USE Massage the lower abdomen with the oil when experiencing period pains. Repeat as often as needed up to 6 times a day.

STORAGE The infused oil and rub will keep for up to 1 year.

VARIATION GINGER AND PEPPER RUB

This rub is more strongly pain-relieving due to the deep-heat properties of the black pepper and ginger, which invigorate circulation to the area. To make the infused oil, use 15g ginger, 2 tsp peppercorns, 10–15g rosemary leaves and 100ml olive or almond oil (follow the recipe above). Use as directed above. Wash hands after use.

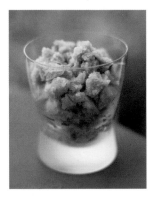

Willow and Lime Pain-Relieving Granita

Willow bark has a wonderful deep, dark, smoky flavour, but more excitingly it also contains salicin, a substance very similar to aspirin. Here I've combined it with lime in a uniquely flavoured, pain-relieving granita – friends say it tastes like everything from Seville orange marmalade to Imperial Leather soap and even chorizo, so take your pick! The granita is slightly slower acting than popping a pill, but its effects should last longer, and it's gentler on the stomach.

2 litres water

40g dried willow bark (*Salix*)

300g sugar (or to taste)

zest and juice of 3 limes

2 tbsp orange blossom water

1 In a pan, pour the freshly boiled water over the dried willow bark and simmer for 10 minutes.

2 Strain out the bark and return the decoction to the pan, simmering uncovered until reduced to about 600ml (about 20–30 minutes). At this stage the mixture will be intensely bitter, but do not let that faze you; sugar and limes can mask a multitude of sins.

3 Take off the heat and stir in the sugar, lime juice, zest and orange blossom water, and leave to cool. Once cool, place in a covered ice cream tray and freeze. This makes about 8 doses.

USE For adults, to relieve the pain of headache, place about 100ml (an ice-cream-scoop-sized dose) in a bowl and eat with a spoon, up to 3 times a day.

CAUTION Anyone who is allergic to aspirin or any other anti-inflammatory drug, or who suffers from an ulcer or has asthma, should not take willow bark. Do not take if you have been warned not to take aspirin by your doctor, or if you are pregnant or breastfeeding. Children and adolescents under 16 years should not take willow bark either. If you are taking any other medication, check with your doctor or pharmacist first.

STORAGE Will keep for up to 1 year in a freezer.

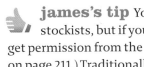 **james's tip** You can buy dried willow bark from most herbal stockists, but if you do want to source the material yourself, be sure to get permission from the landowner first! (See my foraging dos and don'ts on page 211.) Traditionally, it's the inner part of the bark from branches over 5 years old which are believed to be the most potent.

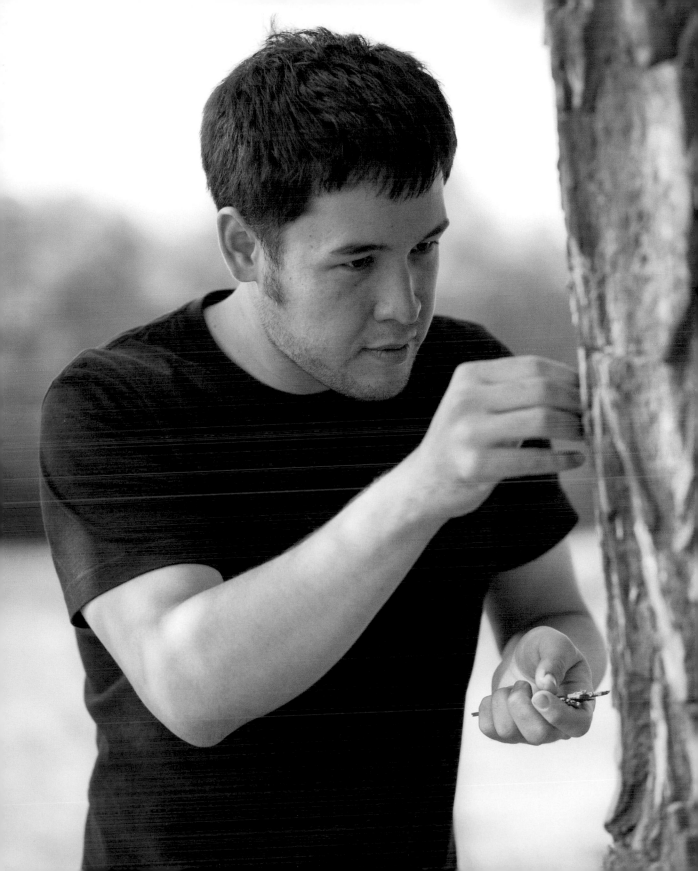

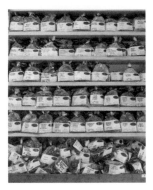

Stress-Proofing Herbal Chai Tea

A twist on the traditional chai recipe, with chamomile and other herbs to help you unwind and relax, and ginseng and fresh ginger to perk you up again when you need it.

I tsp dried Siberian
  ginseng root,
  finely chopped

I tsp coriander seeds

⅛ tsp cinnamon

⅛ tsp cardamom

a pinch of allspice (also
  known as Pimento)

3 tsp fresh ginger root,
  grated

a mugful of water
  or milk

2 tsp German
  chamomile
  (*Matricaria recutita*)

1 Combine everything except the chamomile in a pan and simmer for 20 minutes.

2 Remove from the heat and add the chamomile. Steep for another 10 minutes. Strain the herbs and serve hot. Add milk and/or honey to taste.

USE Drink at once – have 2 or 3 cups daily when you're feeling stressed.

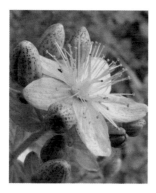

Three Herb Uplift Tea

A good tea to drink if you're feeling low, or as a Seasonal Affective Disorder (SAD) mood-enhancer during dark winter months. St John's wort is highly effective in mild to moderate depression, and lemon balm and lime flowers can help lift the spirits.

50g St John's wort, dried

50g lemon balm flowering tops or leaves, dried

50g lime (linden) flowers (*Tilia* spp.), dried

honey, to taste

lemon juice, to taste

1 Mix the dried plants together, and store in an airtight tin.

2 To make a cup of tea, place 2 teaspoons of Uplift Tea in a mug, pour over freshly boiled water, and leave to infuse for 10 minutes. Strain, then add honey and lemon juice to taste.

USE Drink several times daily, as required.

CAUTION St John's wort can interact with some medicines (especially warfarin). Do not take if you are on any other medication, including the contraceptive Pill, without checking first with your doctor or pharmacist. St John's wort can also increase sensitivity to the sun. Do not use during pregnancy.

STORAGE The dried tea will keep for up to 1 year in an airtight tin.

VARIATION TEA TO LIFT THE SPIRITS

For a wonderfully flavoursome brew, mix together 30g dried lemon balm leaves, 30g dried vervain leaves, 20g dried lavender flowers and 10g dried rose petals (use only those with a good scent), then store in an airtight container. Make freshly before use, by infusing 2 teaspoons tea in a mug of freshly boiled water as above. Cover and leave to infuse for 10 minutes. Drink several times daily, as required. Do not use during pregnancy.

gifting Pack the Uplift Teas into paper or cellophane loose tea packaging or tea storage canisters/caddies (both available from specialist tea/coffee shops). Labelled, these make an unusual home-made gift.

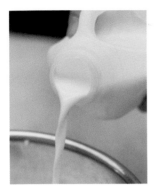

Relaxing Lettuce and Cardamom Milk

Wild lettuce has traditionally been used for its soporific effects – this makes a warming and soothing bedtime drink. I know it sounds like a strange flavour combination, but trust me, it really does work.

6–8 wild lettuce (*Lactuca virosa*) leaves or 3–4 salad lettuce (Cos) leaves

2 cardamom pods

sprinkling grated nutmeg

300ml milk

honey or sugar, to taste

1 Roughly shred the lettuce leaves. Split open the cardamom pods.

2 Place the lettuce, cardamom, grated nutmeg and milk in a pan, and heat gently. Sweeten to taste with honey or sugar.

USE Best drunk warm before bed. If you are drowsy next day, avoid driving or using machinery.

STORAGE Drink as soon as it is made because it will not keep.

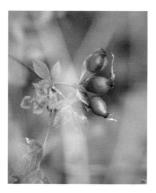

Rosehip and Ginger Fizzy Sherbet

An effervescent hangover remedy based on the World Health Organization's formula for rehydration salts, and containing rosehips for vitamin C and ginger for its anti-sickness effects. The bicarbonate of soda also neutralizes stomach acids to help soothe an irritated, post-boozy tummy. This makes enough for two drinks. Citric acid can be bought from pharmacies.

50g fresh rosehips

1 tsp Maldon salt

2 tsp dried
ground ginger

1 tsp citric acid

2 tsp bicarbonate
of soda

3 tbsp glucose

1 Preheat the oven to 80°C (180°F) or its lowest setting.

2 Bash the rosehips in a mortar and pestle to break them up slightly. This will split the fruit – remove the seeds and discard.

3 Add the salt to the split hips and give them another quick bash with the pestle. The goal is just to break them up a little, not turn them into mush. Scatter the rosehips on a baking tray and put in the oven. Immediately turn off the heat and leave in the oven for 90 minutes.

4 Remove the dried hips from the oven and grind to a fine powder in a spice grinder. Mix with all other ingredients, then store in an airtight container.

USE Add half of the sherbet to 1 litre warm water. Stir and drink freely.

STORAGE Provided it is completely dry, this will keep in an airtight container in a cool, dark place for up to 6 months.

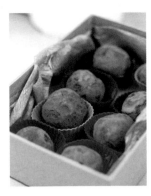

Paraguay Holly and Chilli Truffles

This is a modern take on an original Aztec chocolate recipe! Yerba mate is a stimulating tea made from the leaves of the Paraguay holly tree, and contains caffeine and theobromine. Here, I've mixed it with chilli, vanilla and dark chocolate. These exotic truffles will give you a lift when you're feeling tired. Alternatively, just enjoy them as a tastebud-tingling Christmas treat.

2 medium dried chillies or ½ tsp ground chilli flakes

1 vanilla pod, split in half

1 whole allspice

3 tbsp eucalyptus honey

50g yerba mate (*Ilex paraguariensis*) tea leaves

1 litre boiling water

200g dark chocolate (85% cocoa solids)

3 tsp soft brown sugar

1 tsp cocoa powder

1 Mix the chilli, vanilla pod, allspice and honey together in pan, then add the yerba mate and boiling water. Simmer until the liquid reduces to approximately 150ml – this will take about 45 minutes. Strain and leave to cool to room temperature.

2 Put the chocolate in a glass heatproof bowl, and melt over a pan of hot water.

3 Stir the cooled mate mixture into the melted chocolate, then refrigerate until it takes on a fudge-like consistency (about 30 minutes).

4 Mix the soft brown sugar and cocoa powder in a shallow bowl. Scoop a teaspoon of the truffle mixture and roll into a small ball, then roll in the sugar/cocoa powder to coat. Place each coated truffle in a small paper case. Repeat until all the mixture is used.

USE This one is mainly for adults, because of the caffeine, but you can let older children have one or two! Don't eat more than 6 a day.

CAUTION Contains caffeine.

STORAGE Keep in the refrigerator. Eat within 1 week.

gifting These rich, tangy truffles make a delicious seasonal gift for chocolate fans (that's most of us!). Place them in small silver or gold foil cases, pack in a pretty box, then label and tie with a big ribbon bow – and don't forget to tell the lucky recipient not to eat them all at once.

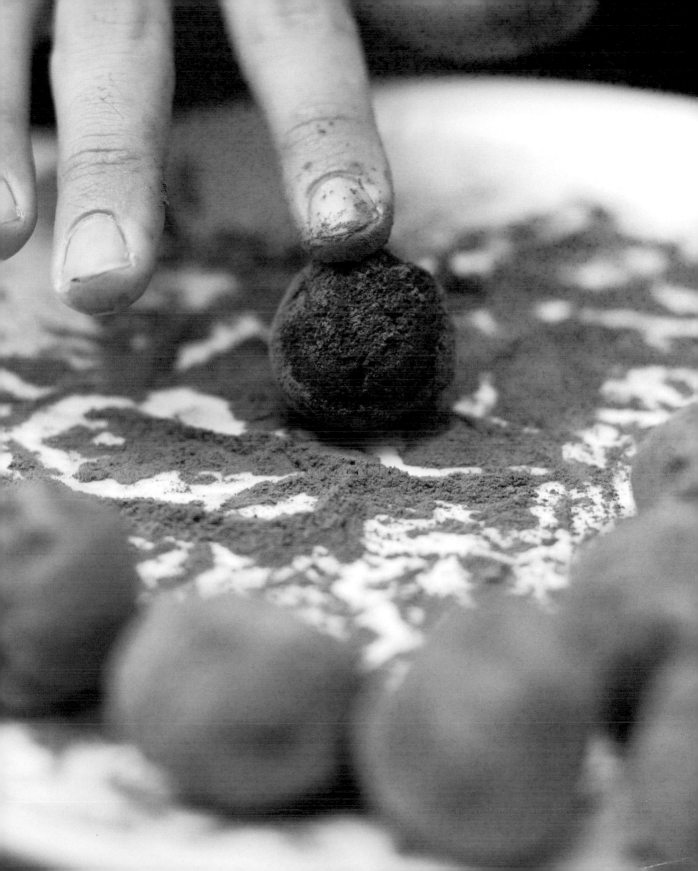

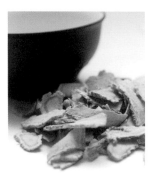

Three Root Syrup Overall Tonic

A tonic to give you an all-round boost: rose root can alleviate low mood and improve physical and mental performance; angelica is traditionally used to aid digestion and soothe coughs and colds; and elecampane is used to treat a range of lung complaints from coughs to bronchitis.

50g rose root (*Rhodiola rosea*)

25g angelica root

25g elecampane root

500ml water

100g brown sugar (per 100ml decoction, see below)

15ml vodka, whisky or brandy (per 100ml decoction, see below)

1 Wash the roots, then boil them in the water for 30 minutes to make a decoction.

2 Strain and measure the liquid into a pan, adding 100g sugar for each 100ml root decoction. Stir, then simmer for 10 minutes.

3 Allow to cool slightly, then measure the liquid again, adding 15ml alcohol per 100ml syrup, to act as a preservative. Bottle and label.

USE Take 1 tablespoon twice daily, one in the morning and one after lunch.

CAUTION Contains alcohol.

STORAGE Will keep for 6 months before opening. Keep in the refrigerator once opened.

gifting This is the perfect gift for anyone you know who suffers from Seasonal Affective Disorder (SAD) or low moods in winter. Just pour into a beautiful bottle, and label with dosage and date.

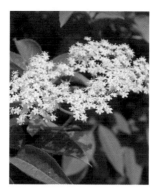

Elderflower 'Champagne'

This is a wonderful elderflower champagne recipe, although you can never be sure from year to year whether it will fizz – it's not fail-safe! If the champagne is flat, add ½ teaspoon of brewer's yeast to each bottle and leave for a further 2 weeks. I don't make huge health claims for this champagne (though elderflowers are traditionally used to soothe symptoms of colds and flu); it's just a delicious, refreshing summer drink and herbal pick-me-up.

3 large elderflower heads

I lemon

750g white or golden sugar

2 tbsp white wine vinegar

4.5 litres water (spring water to be really tasty)

1 Trim the elderflowers from their stems, and gently shake to get rid of any bugs. Zest the lemon and chop the rind finely, then squeeze the juice. Put the elderflowers, lemon rind and juice, sugar, vinegar and water into an earthenware/plastic pot (don't use a metal pan or container). Cover with a cloth or tea towel and leave to steep for 48 hours.

2 Strain the champagne into strong, sterilized screw-top bottles or old-fashioned swing-top bottles (you can reuse some beer or lemonade bottles). Don't use corks or plastic bottles, as they will probably explode.

USE Drink freely as required.

CAUTION This can be mildly alcoholic. Keep away from children.

STORAGE Keep bottles in a cool dark place for up to 3 weeks. The champagne doesn't keep once the bottle is opened – it loses its fizz.

gifting Beautifully bottled and labelled, this makes a great thank-you gift to take to parties.

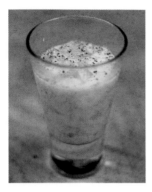

Saffron Egg Nog

East-meets-West in this sweet and warming version of a traditional Christmas drink – saffron is often used in Asian medicine to help soothe anxiety and depression. This makes 6 egg nogs; store it in the refrigerator and drink not more than one shot daily, as a delicious seasonal pick-me-up.

500ml whole milk

2 bay leaves

36 threads/3 pinches saffron

2 strips orange rind

3 tbsp golden syrup

200ml single cream

3 eggs

150ml white rum

grated fresh nutmeg, to serve

1 Pour the milk, bay leaves, saffron, orange rind, golden syrup and cream into a pan, and simmer gently for 10 minutes. Strain through a sieve.

2 Break the eggs into a glass heatproof bowl, then slowly whisk in the hot milk mixture.

3 Place the bowl above a pan of boiling water and heat gently, stirring, until the mixture thickens to a custardy consistency. Then take it straight off the heat.

4 Whisk in the rum, then pour the mixture into a jug. Cool, then leave to stand in the refrigerator for at least 8 hours before serving.

5 Serve over ice with grated nutmeg.

USE Drink no more than 1 wine glass a day.

CAUTION Contains alcohol.

STORAGE Keep in the refrigerator. Will last for 2 weeks.

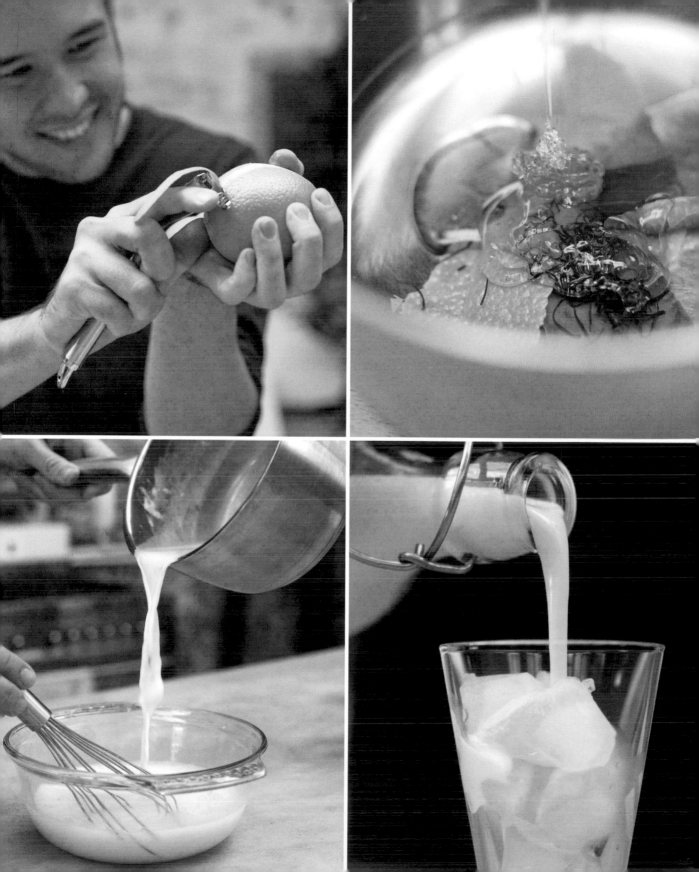

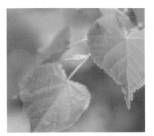

Time of the Month Tea

Drink this relaxing, hormone-balancing brew when you're feeling emotionally wired before or during your period. In summer, you can harvest large quantities of these plants wild or in the garden, and dry them for use over the winter.

30g lady's mantle (*Alchemilla mollis*) leaves

30g lime (linden) flowers (*Tilia* spp.)

15g yarrow flowers

15g skullcap leaves and flowers

750ml water

1 Put all the plants in a glass bowl, and pour over 750ml freshly boiled water. Leave to infuse for 10 minutes. Strain. Drink one cup immediately, then pour the rest into a thermos flask for use throughout the day. This makes enough for 3 mugs or a day's supply.

USE Drink as required, throughout the day.

STORAGE Mix up a large batch of the dried plants and store in a tin, so you can make up the tea as you need it. The dried tea will keep in an airtight container for up to 6 months.

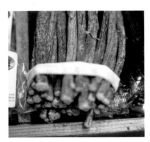

Herbal Elixir for Low Libido

This tonic contains ginseng and damiana – both reputed to have a stimulating, aphrodisiac effect on low libido in men. Hope it works for you!

25g Asian ginseng root (*Panax ginseng*), about 2–3 pieces

50g liquorice root

50g dried damiana leaves (see page 182)

brandy, to cover

black cherry concentrate, from health food stores

honey, optional, to taste

1 Mix the ginseng, liquorice and damiana, then cover completely with brandy and seal in an airtight jar. Leave in a warm, dark place for 7 weeks.

2 Strain, reserving the liquid and the ginseng root.

3 Measure the liquid. For each 250ml liquid, add 125ml black cherry concentrate. Pour into a jar and add the ginseng root. If you like, add some honey to taste, then place the jar in the refrigerator.

USE Take 10ml each night.

CAUTION Contains alcohol. Not to be used with high blood pressure or when in poor health.

STORAGE Keep in the refrigerator and use within 8 weeks.

COSMETIC

Creative head-to-toe botanical beauty treatments and natural health remedies to help pamper, de-stress and nourish body and soul.

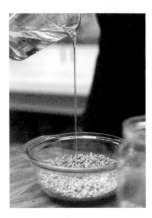

Deep Conditioning Hair Oil

Shampoos can strip the natural oils from the hair and scalp, leaving hair dull and brittle and creating an over-production of sebum, which then makes hair greasy. Giving your hair an oil treatment once a month will help restore balance, condition and shine. See oil infusion method on page 30.

For blonde hair:

infuse chamomile or mullein flowers into your favourite oil – apricot, almond and olive oil all work well.

For dark hair:

infuse sprigs of rosemary or sage leaves into your favourite oil – try apricot, almond, safflower or olive oil.

For fine hair:

infuse rose petals into your favourite oil, such as apricot, almond or olive oil.

For very dry, damaged hair and dandruff:

use jojoba oil, infusing it for blonde, dark or fine hair as above. The oil leaves a light coating on the hair and is especially useful for dry and damaged hair, dandruff or an irritated dry scalp.

USE Once a month as a deep-conditioning treatment. On dry hair, first massage the oil into the scalp, then cover the hair from root to tip. Tie a plastic bag around hair, then cover with a warmed towel. Leave the oil for a couple of hours to soak through thoroughly.

To wash out, first massage a largish amount of shampoo into the hair from root to tip, wet the hair a little and work it into a lather, then rinse out well with warm water. Repeat if hair still feels very oily.

STORAGE Infused oil will keep in a cool dry place for up to 1 year.

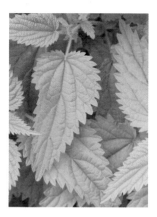

Enriching Hair Treatment Gel

Gel is less messy to use than oil – apply this treatment once or twice a week to help improve scalp condition and leave hair soft and conditioned. Xanthan gum can be bought from health food shops.

Ig or ½ tsp xanthan gum

Choose from the following plants to suit your hair and scalp type:

For dark hair:
use rosemary or sage

For blonde hair:
use chamomile and lime (linden) flowers

For brittle or dry hair and scalp:
use nettles or rose

For dandruff:
use violet/pansy or lady's mantle

For greasy hair:
use yarrow

1 Infuse 2 teaspoons of your chosen plant in a cup of freshly boiled water, and leave covered to steep for 10 minutes.

2 Measure 90ml of the infusion and pour into a bowl.

3 Sprinkle the xanthan gum powder onto the infusion and whisk with an electric hand blender until thickened.

USE Massage directly onto the scalp and hair. Wrap your head in a towel and leave for 30 minutes. Rinse out with warm water or your homemade vinegar rinse. Use once or twice a week.

STORAGE Will keep for a couple of days in the refrigerator, but best made as needed.

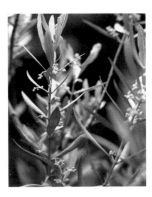

Antioxidant Olive Leaf Clay Mask

Rich in minerals, antioxidants and anti-inflammatories, this soothing mask helps remove dead skin cells and stimulate circulation, leaving skin feeling toned and super soft. Clay powder is available online. See Stockists on page 215.

3–4 heaped tbsp fresh or dried olive leaves

boiling water, to cover

4 tbsp clay powder

14 drops lemon essential oil

1 Place the olive leaves in a pan, pour boiling water over to cover and simmer gently for 10 minutes.

2 Strain out the leaves and return the liquid to the heat, continuing to simmer until reduced by half (about 10 minutes). Measure out 80ml of the olive water.

3 Put the clay powder in a bowl. Pour the olive water slowly over the clay powder, stirring well, then stir in the lemon essential oil. Bottle.

USE When cool, apply the mask to your face, avoiding the eye area. Leave on for 20 minutes, then wash off with warm water. The mask can be applied once or twice a week, as needed. Wash off immediately if you get any redness or irritation.

STORAGE Will keep for 6 months in the refrigerator.

'Now I'm looking at this, I'm starting to feel more and more ripped off with the products I've spent money on because it looks exactly the same...My flatmate tried it and noticed that her chin isn't so red – I'm not sure whether it's a coincidence. Your skin does feel soft like you've moisturized. It's quite a good bargain.' Elena

james's tip You can customize this face mask to suit your skin type. Add ½ teaspoon olive oil along with the lemon essential oil to enrich normal or dry skin; or ½ teaspoon witch hazel for greasy or acne-prone skins.

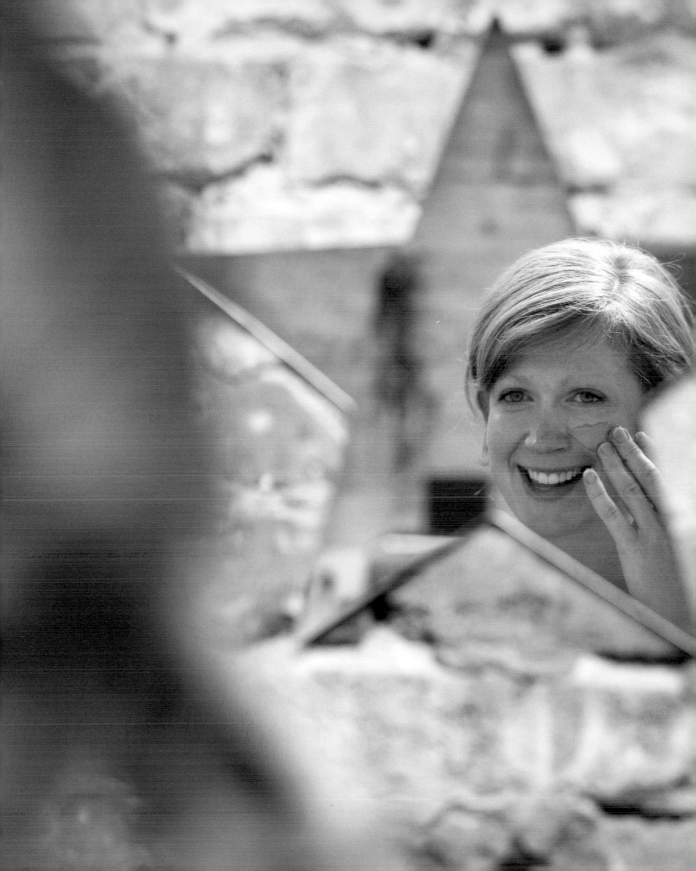

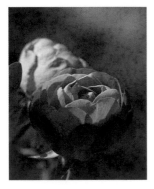

Herbal Vinegar Hair Rinse

Play around with the following plants and aromas to create your own perfect hair rinse – it'll eliminate residual shampoo, help restore the natural acid balance of the scalp, and leave your hair looking clean, soft and incredibly shiny.

Prepare your vinegar (see recipe for base vinegar on page 31), then infuse with the appropriate plant for your hair type (again following the directions on page 31). Try:

chamomile or marigold for fair hair (and irritated scalp)

sage or rosemary for dark hair

nettle, to strengthen brittle hair

violet, marigold or parsley for dandruff

rose petals for dry scalp

for a scented rinse, use rose petals, lavender, lemon balm or jasmine flowers

1 Be creative and add more than one plant, and remember always to use enough vinegar to cover comfortably the plants you are using.

USE Pour a cupful of your vinegar (more if you have long hair) into a jug, dilute with warm water, and use as a final rinse after washing your hair.

STORAGE The infused vinegars will last for up to 1 year.

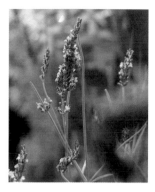

Anti-Dandruff Hair Oil

Rub this sweet-smelling, anti-dandruff oil into the scalp as a pre-conditioning treatment before washing hair. Its antiseptic and anti-inflammatory properties will help soothe and tone a dry, irritated scalp. Use 3 times a week for 2 weeks to blitz dandruff, then once a week to keep it at bay.

6 tbsp fresh rosemary

3 tbsp fresh thyme

3 tbsp fresh lavender

250ml coconut oil

20 drops peppermint essential oil

1 Wash and chop all the plants and place in a glass heatproof bowl. Stir in the coconut oil. Cover the bowl with a lid and place over a pan of boiling water to create a double boiler. Heat on a medium to low flame for 1 hour. Leave to cool.

2 When cool, stir in the peppermint essential oil. Strain and pour the hair oil into bottles.

USE Apply 3 teaspoons to hair and massage well into the scalp. Wrap hair in a towel and leave for 30 minutes. Then wash hair a couple of times with normal shampoo to get the oil out completely. Use 3 times a week for the first 2 weeks, and once a week as a preventative measure.

CAUTION Avoid the eye area, and if you feel any discomfort, wash off immediately.

STORAGE Will keep for up to 1 year in a cool, dark place.

'It smells quite nice, it's got an oily texture. With the exception of thyme I think everything grows in my garden, which is great.' Robert

'It hasn't got rid of the dandruff completely, but I've started to see an improvement where it is starting to lessen, and it's something I've started to mention to my friends.' Neusa

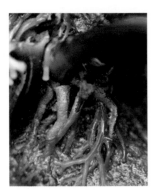

Seaweed and Sand Body Scrub

An easy way to bring a summer holiday vibe into your life this winter – you can pick half these ingredients up off the beach or buy easily online! The carrageen and kelp are packed with nutrients, and the salt and sand are powerful exfoliators, sloughing off dead cells to leave skin feeling soft and looking clear and bright.

25g dried kelp

25g dried carrageen

1.5 litres water

3 large tbsp sea salt

10 tbsp fine, dry beach sand (not builder's sand!)

15 drops rosemary essential oil

1 Soak the kelp and carrageen overnight in the water.

2 Next day, roughly cut the kelp with scissors into small pieces. Place the kelp, carrageen and water mixture in a pan, bring to the boil and simmer for approximately 30 minutes.

3 Place in a blender and whizz. Return the pulp to the pan and heat for 10 minutes more. Stir in the salt, sand and essential oil. Bottle in a glass jar.

USE Gently rub a handful of the scrub over skin in the shower, using circular movements and paying particular attention to rough skin on the knees, feet and elbows. Rinse off well.

CAUTION Do not use on the face. This is quite an abrasive exfoliator, so use no more than once a week.

STORAGE Will keep for 6 months in the refrigerator.

'I was sceptical but the body scrub felt really amazing on my skin – it left it really soft. The only thing is that there was loads of sand in my shower that it took me ages to get rid of!' Karen

> **james's tip** You can pick fresh kelp and carrageen off the beach – they grow prolifically, especially around the west coast of Britain. I'd treat them just as you would if you were going to eat them – make sure the piece has been freshly washed up and is not unusually smelly or full of bugs.
>
> Use about 100g of each, and don't worry about soaking it overnight – just add enough water to bring the volume to 1.5 litres and follow the recipe from Step 2 above.
>
> Take along a bucket and bring home some clean, fine sand too (enough to fill a child's small beach bucket by one-third). Sand is a constantly renewed resource and you're taking a tiny amount, but check before harvesting seaweed or sand with your local authority that looks after the beach (you'll find them on www.direct.gov.uk).

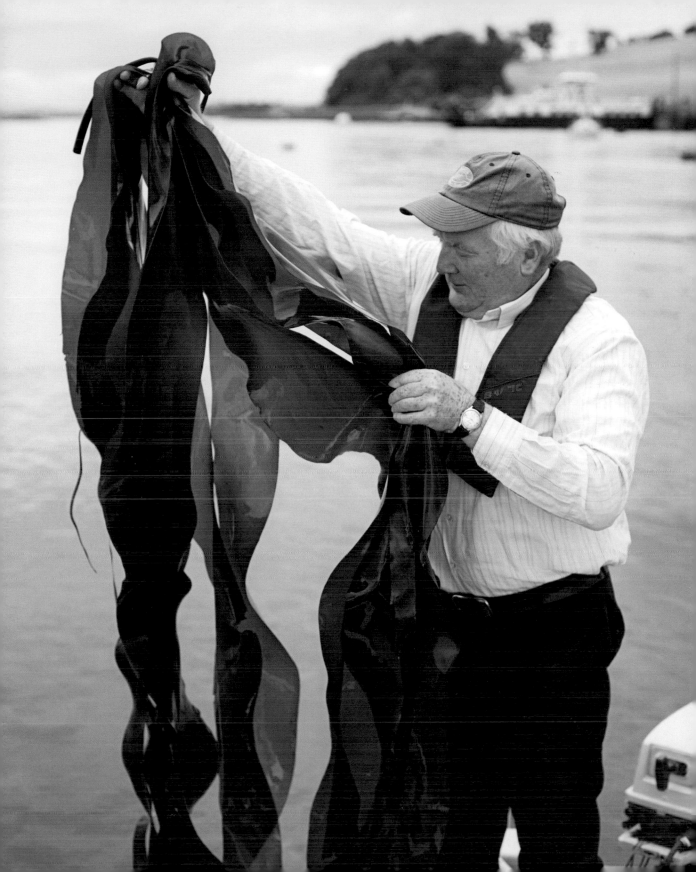

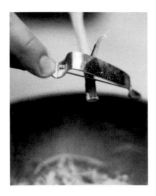

Green Tea, Liquorice and Lemon Mouthwash

Liquorice roots have an intensely sweet flavour, yet they don't contain any actual sugar, and are actually good for teeth, helping to slow the growth of bacteria and formation of plaque. Green tea inhibits the bacteria responsible for mouth odour, and both are anti-inflammatory, soothing sore gums. Use this mouthwash once a day to help freshen breath and help keep tooth decay at bay.

For the tincture:

2 liquorice sticks

5 tsp green tea leaves

about 200ml vodka, or to cover

For the mouthwash:

2–4 tsp green tea leaves

8 drops lemon essential oil

1 tsp glycerine

'In terms of taste and freshness and feeling clean, I'm pleasantly surprised. I will finish the bottle off and I would try it again.' Steve

To make the tincture:
Peel the liquorice into shavings as you would a carrot, using a very sharp vegetable peeler (but see Tip below). Combine with the first quantity of tea leaves (5 tsp) in a glass jar. Add enough vodka to cover the herbs completely. Cover and keep in a cool dark place for 10–14 days. Then strain the mixture, reserving the liquid.

To make the mouthwash:
Using 2–4 tsp green tea leaves, make up a pot of green tea and leave to stand for 2–3 minutes. Strain a 200ml measure of the green tea, then pour this into the liquorice tincture to dilute it. (When you do this, the tea should be no hotter than 80–90°C/176–194°F – definitely not boiling.) Stir in the lemon essential oil and glycerine and bottle.

USE Use as a mouthwash/gargle once a day as needed. Do not swallow.

CAUTION Contains alcohol.

STORAGE Will keep for 6 months in the refrigerator.

james's tip There should be a health warning on this recipe: liquorice can ruin your peeler! It's tough stuff, and unless your vegetable peeler is incredibly sharp, you're better off scraping the liquorice root with a sharp knife or bashing it with a pestle on a chopping board. The flavour is so strong that when you're cutting it you seem to be able to taste its intense sweetness at the back of your throat and – even more weirdly – inside your nose ...

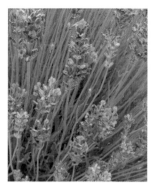

Eau de Cologne

A DIY cologne to splash all over. I use full-strength vodka and fresh herbs to capture the essential oils that provide the main aromas. You can create your own signature scent by playing around with different amounts and combinations of the herbs below. Remember to write down the mix so you can make it again.

For the base, try handfuls of:

eau de cologne mint (*Mentha x piperita f. citrata*) or any mint you like

lavender

lemon balm

peel of ¼ lemon or ¼ orange (or use both If you like a pungent citrus smell)

Other herbs you can add:

basil, bay, rosemary, sage, thyme

Spices you can add (optional):

aniseed, caraway, cardamom, cinnamon

You'll also need:

enough vodka (80% proof or 40% alcohol) to cover

1 Bruise or roughly chop the mint, lavender and lemon balm, along with your choice of other herbs, then add the lemon and/or orange peel and place in a wide-mouthed jar. Cover with the vodka and seal. Leave in a warm (but not hot) place for 12 hours or overnight. This is long enough to capture the volatile oils, but not the tannins.

2 Next day, strain and then leave the infused vodka to 'mature' like a perfume for a further 2 weeks before making a decision about the scent. You may then want to add some more herbs and leave to infuse for another 12 hours or overnight as before. Strain again.

3 Spices add deeper notes and, if you wish to add them, these can be infused now. Add them in small amounts. Spices should be left in the vodka for 2 weeks before straining again.

4 Once you're happy with the scent, decant into small spray bottles.

USE Spray on as required.

STORAGE Will keep for up to 1 year.

gifting Experiment to find an aroma that you think will appeal particularly to your partner or friend. Then bottle in a gorgeous old perfume or spray bottle (you can pick them up cheap in second-hand shops), give the eau de cologne a creative name, label – and you have a truly personal gift from the heart.

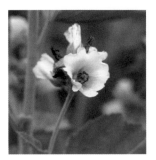

Marshmallow Leaf and Flower Milk Bath for Dry Skin

The milk draws out the softening mucilaginous qualities in both marshmallow and oats, to make a soothing, moisturizing bath for those with dry or sensitive skin.

12–15 heaped tbsp marshmallow leaves and flowers, bruised and sliced

2–3 tbsp oats

boiling water, to cover

250–500ml milk

1 Place the marshmallow leaves and flowers and the oats in a saucepan and add enough freshly boiled water to cover. Place a lid over the pan and leave for 10 minutes to steep.

2 Use a potato masher to squash the leaves in the pan so that they release the gooey mucilage.

3 Add the milk to the marshmallow goo, then gently heat through. Strain the mixture and add to a hot bath.

USE Enjoy a long soak in the bath, no need to wash off.

STORAGE This won't keep, so make it as you need it.

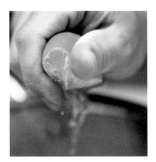

Yogurt, Lime and Strawberry Face Pack

The lime and strawberry contain alpha hydroxy fruit acids that naturally exfoliate while the yogurt nourishes, leaving skin feeling smooth and soft. Makes enough for 1 face mask.

5 strawberries (or 20 wild strawberries)

small pot of natural yogurt

juice of ¼ lime

1 tbsp oat bran

1 Blend the strawberries with the yogurt and lime juice. Stir in the oat bran ½ teaspoon at a time, until the mixture thickens slightly. Apply to clean skin, avoiding the eye area. Leave on for 30 minutes.

2 Wash off with warm water and a flannel or damp towel.

USE Most effective when used immediately.

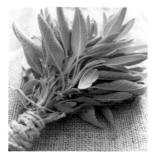

Bicarb, Myrrh and Sage Tooth Whitening Powder

Bicarbonate of soda is a gentle but effective abrasive to clean teeth and gums, sage has long been used to whiten teeth (a fresh leaf rubbed on the teeth is an old whitening remedy) and myrrh resin has a history of use as an oral antiseptic and breath-freshener.

1½ tbsp sage leaves, dried

10g myrrh resin

200g bicarbonate of soda

1 Pound together the sage leaves and myrrh resin in a mortar and pestle until finely ground. Add the bicarbonate of soda and mix together. Store in a shallow, wide-mouthed jar with a lid to keep airtight.

USE Dip a slightly moistened toothbrush in the powder and brush teeth, rinse and spit.

STORAGE Will keep in an airtight container for up to 1 year.

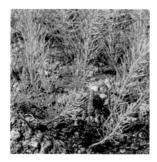

Horsetail and Celery Seed Nail Bath

Horsetail contains silicic acid and flavonoids, which help boost healing, and has traditionally been used as a wound healer and to strengthen weak and brittle nails. This easy-to-make nail bath can be used on toenails too.

30g horsetail (*Equisetum arvense*)

30g celery seeds

220ml water

1 Put the chopped horsetail and celery seeds in a bowl. Pour 220ml freshly boiled water over and leave to stand for 1 hour. Strain the liquid and store in a wide-necked jar.

USE Each day, warm the liquid, and soak fingernails (or toenails) for 10 minutes.

STORAGE Make a fresh batch every 3 days.

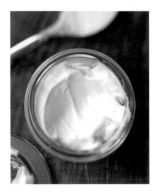

Oats and Almond Moisturizing Body Cream

This rich, soothing cream is full of nourishing ingredients that help skin retain moisture and stay smooth and supple. Good for dry and mature skins.

300ml water

2 tbsp rolled oats

2 tsp beeswax

6 tsp emulsifying wax

40ml almond oil

2 tsp honey

2 tsp vitamin C powder

6–12 drops chamomile essential oil (optional)

'I was a bit sceptical of whether it would work, because I thought it was just going to be the same as every other cream, but it wasn't. The patches of dried skin on my arms have gone down.' Gemma

1 In a pan, heat the water until boiling and then add the oats. Simmer uncovered for 10 minutes. Strain the oats, reserving the liquid into a measuring jug – you need 200ml. Put in a pan and keep hot.

2 Heat the beeswax and emulsifying wax together very gently in another pan with the almond oil until the waxes fully dissolve. Take off the heat and immediately whisk in a little of the hot oat liquid into the wax mixture. Keep adding the hot oat liquid, a little at a time, making sure it is well mixed between additions, until you have used up all 200ml.

3 Stir in the honey and vitamin C powder and, if desired, add in a few drops of chamomile essential oil, which acts as a preservative, is anti-inflammatory and adds a delicious scent. (Don't worry if you don't have chamomile – you can use any essential oil you have around.) Pour the cream into wide-mouthed pots, and seal at once.

USE After bathing, pat skin gently dry, then apply the cream as needed. On tough areas of dry skin such as knees, elbows and feet, use twice daily, especially before bed.

STORAGE Will keep in the refrigerator for up to 1 month.

gifting Give a pot of this rich body cream to friends as a treat in winter when skin needs an extra boost. You can buy gift pots second-hand, from car boot sales or from specialist suppliers (see Stockists, page 215). Just add an ornamental label with the storage details on.

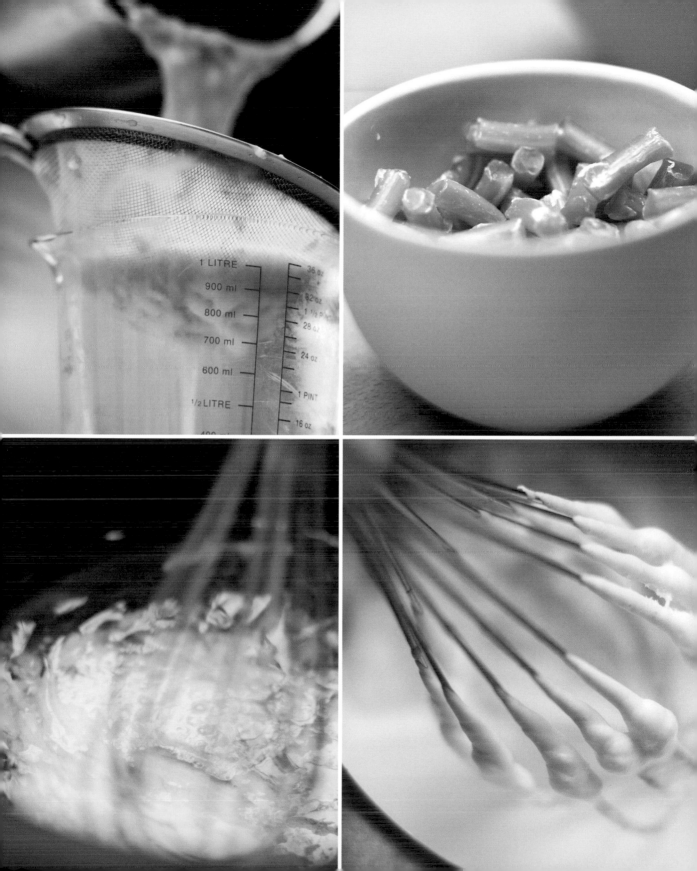

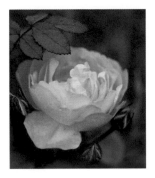

Rose and Clove Hair Removing Sugar

Sugaring is a popular method of hair removal in the Middle East, considered just as effective as, but less painful than, waxing. Here I've added in some cloves for their mild anaesthetic action as well. This rose-infused sugar smells wonderful, is gentle on skin, and is easy to apply and wash off afterwards.

petals of 12 scented
   roses

500g sugar

1 tsp whole cloves

juice of 1½ lemons

2 tbsp rosewater
   (optional, for scent)

cotton or linen cloth,
   cut into strips

1 Wash the rose petals, gently dab dry, then chop them roughly.

2 In a glass jar, layer the sugar with the petals, and leave in a cool, dark place overnight. After 12–24 hours you will have a thick syrup filled with sugar crystals.

3 Pour the rose-infused sugar syrup into a pan. Grind the cloves in a pestle and mortar and add to the mix. Heat for a few minutes on a low heat until the sugar crystals melt and disappear – it should be clear and the colour of the petals.

4 Add the lemon juice and continue on a low heat until the syrup thickens.

5 Strain off the petals through a sieve into a second pan. Heat for 20 minutes, or until the syrup reduces, thickens and turns a dark caramel colour. Take off the heat and add the rosewater, if using, for scent. Bottle in a close-stoppered or sealed container, to stop moisture being absorbed or the sugar crystallizing. Alternatively, cool until lukewarm, then use at once.

USE Use a wooden spreader or palette knife to apply a thin layer of lukewarm sugar (check it's not too hot by doing a small test patch first). Cover the sugared area with a cloth strip, pushing down firmly, then quickly pull the strip away in the opposite direction to the growth of hair. Repeat until all hair is removed. If the sugar cools and becomes too hard to use, gently heat again until lukewarm, then reapply. Wash skin in lukewarm water after sugaring, to remove any residue.

NB If you have sensitive skin, you can reduce irritation by pulling off the sugar in the direction of hair growth.

CAUTION Don't use on highly sensitive, broken or sunburned skin, in cases of eczema or psoriasis, or on hairs growing from moles or warts. Keep skin out of the sun for 24 hours afterwards.

STORAGE If bottled correctly, this will keep in a cool, dry place for up to 1 year.

james's tip In the interests of science, I tried this on a section of leg hair – it worked brilliantly. But, as with waxing, hair needs to be a certain length first. Some people like to dust their skin lightly with cornflour before sugaring, but you don't have to – sugar doesn't stick to skin in anything like the same way as wax.

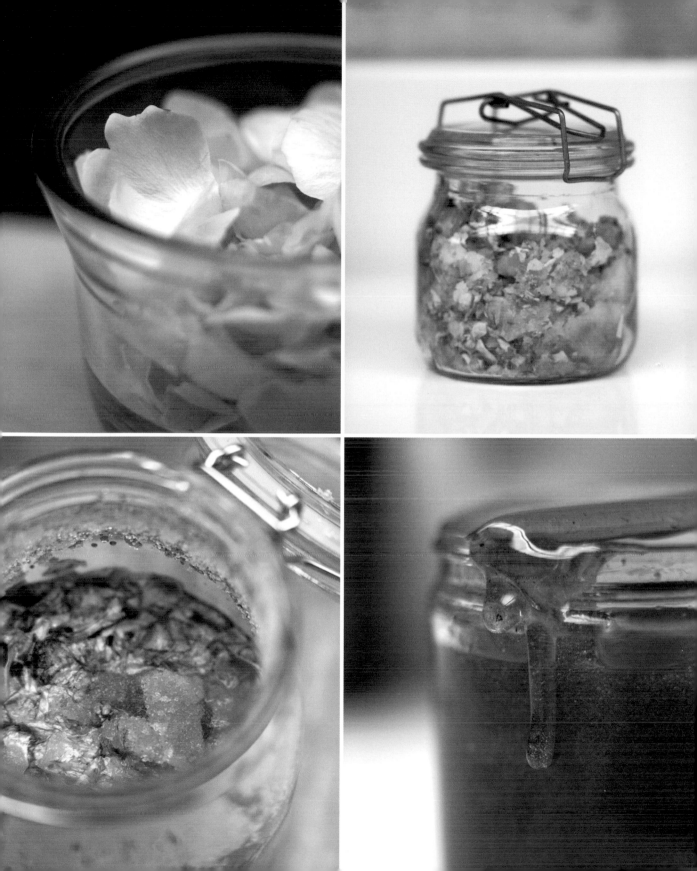

Eyebright Compress

The eyebright and black tea in this refreshing compress contain astringent and anti-inflammatory substances that help soothe, tone and tighten tissues – giving a boost to tired or puffy eyes. Apply to your eyes whenever they need a holiday. To buy empty tea bags, which are ready to be filled, see Stockists, page 215. Alternatively, make your own from muslin.

2 tsp dried eyebright

2 tsp ordinary black tea leaves

2 unfilled tea bags

small amount of hot water

1 Mix the dried eyebright and tea leaves in a small bowl, then spoon into 2 empty tea bags. Seal or fold over the bags. Place the bags in a shot glass of hot but not boiling water. Leave for 10 minutes, then squeeze out and place one over each eye.

USE Relax with the eye compresses on for 10–15 minutes.

STORAGE Make fresh as you need it.

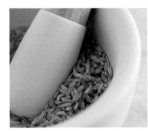

Fennel Seed Eye Bath for Conjunctivitis

A simple recipe traditionally used to treat conjunctivitis and blepharitis, or simply to brighten eyes before a night out.

½ tsp fennel seeds

100ml boiling water

2 eye baths (available cheaply from pharmacies)

1 Place the fennel seeds in a ceramic cup; pour over the boiling water to make an infusion. Cover and leave for 10 minutes. Strain and allow to cool in a covered bowl.

USE Place the cooled infusion in 2 separate eye baths – if using for infection, always use a separate eye bath for each eye, to prevent cross-infection. Place the eye bath over the infected eye and bathe for around a minute, three times daily for infection. To brighten eyes, use about 1 hour before going out.

STORAGE Place any excess in a sterilized bottle and use throughout the day.

VARIATION CORNFLOWER EYE BATH
Cornflowers have a long history of use for tired and sore eyes, with cornflower extracts still popular in France today. Use 1 teaspoon of fresh cornflowers in place of the fennel in the recipe above.

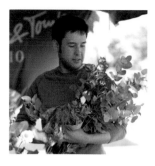

Sugar Body Scrub

Once you've infused a batch of oil with your favourite plant, you can use it both for the Deep Conditioning Hair Oil (see page 120) and as the base in this rich, moisturizing body scrub. For the infused oil, see the recipe on page 30. Using castor oil, makes the scrub more spreadable and also draws out impurities.

100g brown sugar

5ml safflower oil

18ml infused oil of your choice: rose petals for mature skin, marigold (*Calendula officinalis*) for normal skin, chickweed for dry skin, chamomile for sensitive skin

5ml castor oil

20–25 drops essential oils – choose any scents you like

1 Mix all the ingredients together and place in a wide-mouthed jar.

USE Shower first with warm water, then work handfuls of scrub into the skin using circular movements. Rinse off well.

STORAGE Will keep for 1 year.

gifting This Sugar Body Scrub makes a glamorous and useful Christmas or birthday present. Create an infused oil that suits the person's skin, then add the ingredients as above, and bottle in a beautiful glass jar with a hand-penned label.

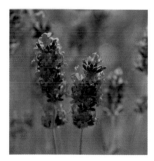

Roman Chamomile and Lavender Acne Steam

A very simple treatment for acne, which encourages the softening of blocked pores and helps bring spots to a head. Both chamomile and lavender have anti-inflammatory and antiseptic properties, to cleanse and soothe inflamed skin.

a bowl of boiling water

3 tbsp Roman chamomile (*Anthemis nobilis*) flowers, fresh or dried

3 tbsp lavender flowers, fresh or dried

1 Fill a glass or plastic bowl with freshly boiled water. Add the chamomile and lavender flowers.

USE Lean your face over the bowl and create a closed environment by putting a towel around the back of your head and over the bowl – be very careful to remain at least 30cm above the hot water. Steam for 5–10 minutes, then gently pat your face dry – do not rub. Steam daily for acne.

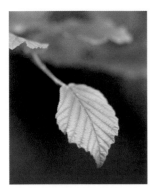

Witch Hazel Aftershave Gel for Shaving Rash

This is a proper old-school aftershave, the kind used by barbers with a red and white pole outside their shops. It combines witch hazel tincture with witch hazel water for maximum effect. Rub on after shaving – it smells fantastic, and the witch hazel can help prevent infection, tighten pores and soothe skin.

To make the witch hazel tincture:

50g fresh witch hazel leaves and twigs, or 25g dried

zest of 4 limes

10 bay leaves

10 scented pelargonium 'Old Spice' leaves

about 450ml white rum (40% alcohol or 80% proof), to cover

To make the witch hazel water:

50g fresh witch hazel leaves and twigs

1 litre of water

To make the aftershave gel:

4 sachets vegetable gelatine

To make the witch hazel tincture:
Chop the witch hazel leaves and twigs and place in a jar with the lime zest, bay leaves and 'Old Spice' pelargonium leaves. Pour the rum over to cover and store in a cool, dark place for 10 days to 1 month, shaking the tincture every couple of days.

To make the witch hazel water:
Put the chopped witch hazel leaves and twigs into a pan, cover with the water and simmer gently for 1 hour or so, reducing the liquid until you have 100ml left. Strain.

To make the aftershave gel:
When the tincture has infused for 10 days to 1 month, strain and measure 200ml into a pan. Add 100ml of the witch hazel water, then mix in 4 sachets of vegetable gelatine. Place the pan on a low heat, whisking as it thickens. Once thick, take off the heat, and bottle.

USE Splash on after shaving, as needed.

STORAGE The gel will keep for 4 weeks in the refrigerator. The tincture will keep for at least 1 year.

The skin's calming down, there's no redness there, the bleeding's almost stopped, there's one or two spots. It works really well and smells really nice.' Nathan

'It does have a positive effect, but shaving every day and passing a blade over my skin every day – it just makes the rash too much, and therefore the remedy can't cope.' Simon

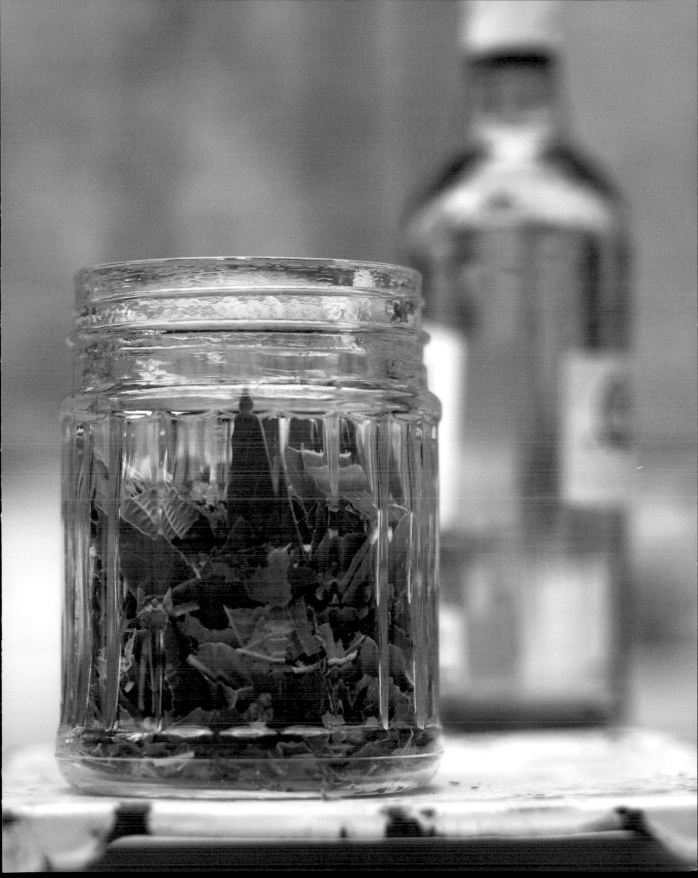

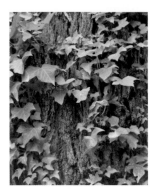

Ivy, Juniper and Grapefruit Cream

Applied externally, ivy is often used as a toning treatment for cellulite. In this rich, moisturizing cream, ivy is mixed with aromatic grapefruit and juniper for their anti-inflammatory effects, to help ease tired and aching legs.

50g fresh ivy leaves (*Hedera helix*)

250ml gin

peel of 2 grapefruit

10 drops juniper essential oil

2 tbsp sunflower oil

3 tsp emulsifying wax

1 tsp beeswax

1 Preheat the oven to 80°C (180°F) or its lowest setting.

2 Wash the ivy leaves, pat dry, and chop roughly. Place on a baking tray and put in the oven for 1 hour.

3 Blitz the dried ivy leaves in a blender with the gin, grapefruit peel and juniper essential oil. Strain through a sieve into a bowl to remove all fibre, squeezing the pulp with your hands to extract as much liquid as possible.

4 Heat the sunflower oil, emulsifying wax and beeswax in a heatproof glass bowl above a pan of boiling water, until all the wax has melted. Take off the heat and slowly whisk in the ivy liquid, 1 tablespoon at a time. Pour into glass jars and leave to cool.

USE Apply to legs once or twice a day for up to 3 weeks. Then take a two-week break before using again.

CAUTION For external use only. Do not use if you are allergic to ivy.

STORAGE Keep in the refrigerator. Use within 2 months.

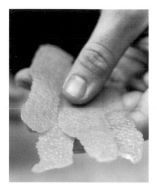

Orange-Scented Body Oil

The fragrance of Christmas – orange, cloves and exotic myrrh – in a bottle. This luxe body oil makes the most of myrrh's anti-inflammatory properties: apply liberally to moisturize and nourish dry skin, or use as a sweet-smelling massage lotion.

peel of 5 oranges
 or tangerines

4 tbsp cloves

400ml sunflower oil

1 tbsp myrrh resin

1 Put the orange peel, cloves and sunflower oil into a blender and whizz until smooth.

2 Pour the mixture into a glass heatproof bowl and place over a pan of boiling water. Add the myrrh, then cover and leave to simmer for 1 hour, making sure the pan does not boil dry.

3 Take off the heat and leave to cool. Strain the mixture and bottle up.

USE Apply as needed to dry skin, or use for massage.

STORAGE Will keep in a cool, dark place for up to 3 months.

 gifting Bottled up in decorative jars and bottles, this oil makes a luxurious seasonal gift. Just add a label with storage details.

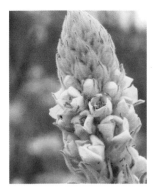

Mullein Ear Drops for Waxy Ears

A build-up of ear wax is normal, especially as you age, but it can be painful and even cause temporary hearing loss. We've put a new twist on this very popular recipe from the last book, using olive oil and adding lavender to the mullein. Used every few months, these drops will help prevent wax from accumulating. Used on problem or compacted wax, they'll soothe pain and dissolve it gently away.

2–3 tbsp fresh or dried mullein flowers

2–3 tbsp fresh or dried lavender flowers, or a few drops of essential oil of lavender

250ml extra virgin olive oil

1 Wash the mullein flowers. Put into a jar with the lavender flowers (if using) and cover with olive oil. Leave to steep for several days in sunlight. Alternatively, if you need to infuse the oil more quickly, place the flowers and olive oil in a small pan and warm on the stove on a very gentle heat for several hours.

2 Strain the infused oil through muslin, add a few drops of lavender essential oil (if using), and filter into sterilized dropper bottles.

USE For adults and children over 2, place 2–3 drops into the affected ear, morning and night, for at least 5 days. The best way to do this is to lie down, sore ear facing up. Gently pull the outer ear backwards, and drop the oil (at room temperature) into the ear canal. Gently massage the area in front of the ear to encourage the oil to flow into the ear canal. Remain lying down for a few minutes. When you stand up, wipe any excess oil with a tissue.

CAUTION If the ear is very painful, discharging matter, or you suspect an ear infection, you must see your doctor. Do not use the drops if you have (or suspect you have) a burst eardrum.

STORAGE Will keep in a cool dark place for 3 months.

james's tip Sometimes you'll find that some tiny bugs are using mullein's bell-shaped flowerheads as a hiding place. If using fresh flowers, soak them well to eradicate any insect life before you start this recipe.

'When I first put the drops in my ears I had an immediate reaction, which was brown liquid coming out of my right ear. I know it doesn't sound pleasant but it was quite pleasing to see that come out! I don't think it's made a huge difference with regards to my hearing but with regards to cleanliness and the potential to get blocked up in the future I think it has made a big difference.' Mark

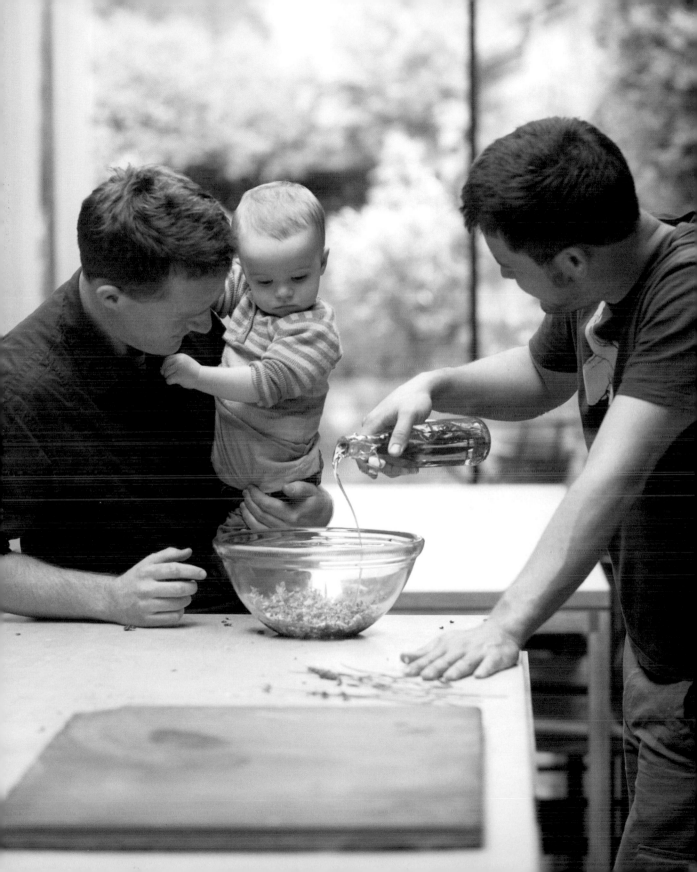

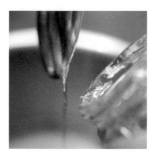

Honey and Yogurt Dry Skin Face Mask

The infused oil soothes and nourishes while the honey yogurt mix leaves skin feeling vibrantly toned and rejuvenated. For the marshmallow leaf infusion, see page 130. For the infused oil, see page 30.

1 tsp honey

2 tsp fresh marshmallow leaf infusion

1 tbsp natural yogurt

1 tbsp brewer's yeast

1 tsp olive oil or infused oil (such as marigold petal or chickweed)

1 Thin down the honey with 2 tsp warm marshmallow leaf infusion, then mix in the yogurt and brewer's yeast until it forms a smooth, thick paste.

USE First spread the olive or infused oil onto clean skin, and then spread the honey yogurt paste on top. Leave for 10–15 minutes, then wash off with tepid water and a flannel or tissues.

STORAGE Make as needed – do not store.

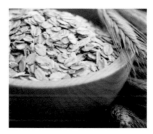

Gardener's Hand Scrub

Honey moisturizes, jojoba oil softens, oatmeal cleanses – just add fresh elderflowers, chamomile or marshmallow to customize this hand scrub to suit your skin type. For the infusion, see the recipe on page 29.

1 tbsp oatmeal or oatbran

1 tsp honey

1 tsp jojoba oil (optional, but good for dry skin)

juice of ¼ lemon

1 tbsp of an infusion of one of the following:

elderflowers, to whiten the hands

chamomile flowers, for sensitive hands

marshmallow leaves, for dry hands

marigold flowers, for chapped hands

1 Mix all the ingredients together, adding a little more lemon juice if the mixture is too dry.

2 Use as a hand scrub, then rinse off with warm water.

USE Makes enough for 1 scrub, best used immediately.

STORAGE This won't keep, so make it up as you need it.

KIDS

Natural, safe and gentle remedies for a wide range of childhood problems from eczema and warts to headlice, upset tummies and wintry sniffles. Get the kids involved making these recipes too: creating their own hands-on remedy is the most exciting introduction to the wonder of plants and science.

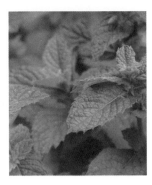

Mint and Chamomile Ice Lollies for Upset Tummies

Ice lollies are a wonderful way to trick unsuspecting children into taking plant remedies, with the combination of mint and chamomile here teaming up to soothe even the most upset of tummies.

40g German chamomile (*Matricaria recutita*)

40g mint (peppermint, catmint or spearmint)

600ml water, freshly boiled

honey, to taste

1 Make a strong herbal tea by putting the chamomile and mint in a bowl and pouring the freshly boiled water over. Leave to infuse for 15–20 minutes for full flavour. Strain into a jug and leave to cool.

2 If you wish to sweeten, add honey to the strained tea, to taste.

3 Leave the tea until cold, then pour into ice-lolly moulds (or make into ice cubes) and put in the freezer.

USE For children over 2, the lollies are soothing to suck on when experiencing an upset tummy. For particularly fussy eaters, the herbal ice-cubes can be snuck into juice, for a home remedy by stealth. Use as often as required.

STORAGE Will keep for up to 3 months in the freezer.

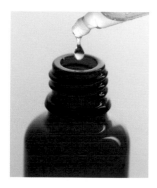

Quassia Head Lice and Nit Treatment

The Caribbean quassia tree, like many other plants, has evolved a range of remarkable insecticidal chemicals to defend itself against millions of years of creepy-crawly attacks. Combined with the essential oils of other like-minded plants, quassia tincture can make a particularly lethal head lice treatment that is nonetheless entirely safe to be used on the non-six-legged among us.

Makes enough for I dose

60ml cider vinegar

20ml quassia tincture (see page 31)

3 drops rosemary essential oil

3 drops lavender essential oil

3 drops eucalyptus essential oil

3 drops tea tree essential oil

I drop anise essential oil

1 Put all the ingredients into a glass jar, then shake well.

USE Apply to dry hair, combing through thoroughly (preferably with a nit comb) and rubbing well into the scalp. Leave in overnight or as long as you like – the treatment is non-greasy so shouldn't need shampooing out for a while. Apply the treatment every couple of days as required, or until all nits are gone.

CAUTION Not to be used on children under 2.

STORAGE Will keep for up to 1 year.

james's tip Unlike many conventional insecticides, the ingredients in this treatment do not just kill adult lice but also penetrate even the waxy protective shields of the hard-to-eradicate eggs, killing the insects before they hatch. Grab your mixing spoon and declare war...

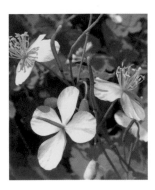

Wart-Fighting Balm

The greater celandine *(Chelidonium majus)* grows easily in the garden, and its leaves and stems are a traditional remedy for warts. In spring and summer, you can rub the bitter-tasting leaves straight on to affected skin, but this celandine wart-fighting balm is handy for all-year-round use. You can find glycerine in most pharmacies.

For the glycerite (infused glycerin), you'll need:

10 heaped tbsp greater celandine leaves and stems (or enough to fill your chosen jar)

about 300ml glycerine, to cover

To make a 30g jar of balm you'll need:

3 dessertspoons celandine-infused glycerine

1½ dessertspoons emulsifying wax

10 drops lemon essential oil

FOR THE GLYCERITE:

1 Put the celandine into a jam jar and cover with the glycerine. Leave for 2 weeks, giving the jar a shake or stir every so often. The glycerine will turn a deep golden colour.

2 Strain the mixture through a sieve or press out through muslin into a bowl. This glycerite forms the basis of the balm below.

NB The glycerite won't keep for more than 1 month.

FOR THE BALM:

1 Put the infused glycerine and wax in a double boiler and heat gently until the wax has completely melted. Take off the heat and beat gently until the balm is smooth and pale. Stir in the lemon essential oil, then pour into a jar and allow to cool completely – the mixture will solidify as it cools.

USE Apply twice daily for several weeks, keeping the area covered with a plaster.

CAUTION Keep away from sensitive areas and healthy skin. Not to be used on children under 2.

STORAGE The balm will keep for up to 1 year.

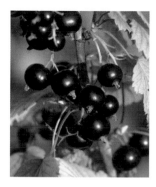

Blackcurrant Tonic

Kids love this rich, fruity syrup that contains anthocyanins, which produce a lovely purple colour and are powerful antioxidants, and there is the added bonus that blackcurrants are rich in vitamin C! Using dried berries makes this syrup a simple way to boost children's fruit intake during autumn and winter. You can pour it over ice-cream and milky puddings too.

250g blackcurrants, dried

500ml distilled water

125ml honey

1 Put the blackcurrants in a pan, add the water and simmer for 15 minutes. Then mash to a pulp with a potato masher. Return the pan to the heat to simmer for another 15 minutes. (Don't heat for too long, to retain as much vitamin C as possible!)

2 Leave the berry mash to cool to room temperature, then strain through muslin. Stir in the honey. Pour into a glass jar and store in the refrigerator.

USE Take 2 teaspoons morning and night. Can be used for adults, and children aged 2 16.

STORAGE Will keep in the refrigerator for up to 2 weeks.

gifting Bottle this up in cute bottles, each with the child's name (and dosage) written on the label, and donate one to each of the children in your life.

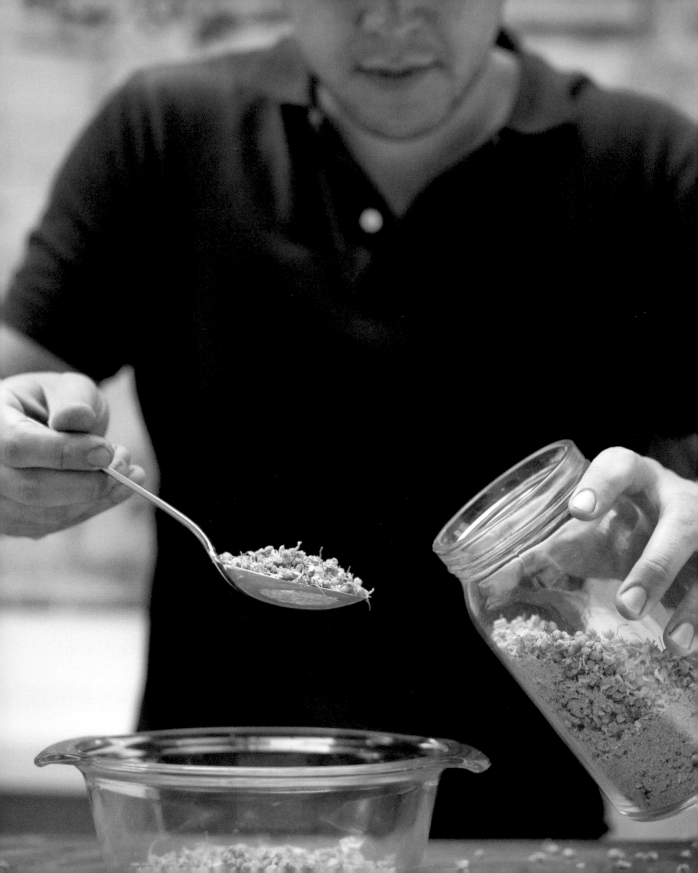

Chamomile Bath Milk

Chamomile's anti-inflammatory and antibacterial properties make it soothing for irritated skin conditions such as psoriasis and eczema, and enriching for dry, itchy or sensitive skins. Normally people add only a small tablespoon-sized splash of bath milk to the tub, which I've always thought is a ridiculously small amount compared with the hundreds of litres of water in the average bath. At such microscopically low concentrations, it is extremely implausible that any of the active chemicals could have any effect whatsoever.

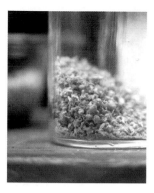

30g dried chamomile flowers (or 60g fresh)

500ml sunflower oil

20 drops lavender essential oil

100ml coconut cream

The great thing about this sunflower oil-based milk, however, is that it's light and non-greasy and also has the benefit of being very cheap, so you can really go crazy and splash in as much as you want for an effective, luxurious and skin-soothing soak.

For the coconut cream, buy either tins or blocks of creamed coconut and follow the instructions to make it up into liquid form.

1 Mix the chamomile flowers and sunflower oil together in a glass heatproof bowl. Cover and place the bowl above a pan of simmering water. Simmer gently for 1 hour, being careful the pan does not boil dry (make sure there is no gap between the pan and bowl), then leave to cool.

2 Once cool, strain the oil and discard the spent flowers. Stir in the lavender essential oil. The resultant chamomile and lavender-scented oil also makes a brilliant soothing skin and massage oil that will keep for up to 1 year.

3 To transform the floral oil into a dispersing bath milk: whisk the oil 1 tablespoon at a time into the coconut cream, making sure the mixture is thoroughly combined between additions of oil. You should end up with a rich milk, about the consistency of double cream. All you've got to do then is bottle it up.

USE Pour 100–200ml of the milk into the bath. Can be used for adults, and children aged 2–16.

STORAGE Keep refrigerated, and use within 1 month.

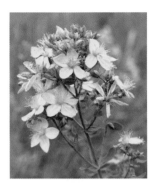

St John's Wort Salve

Its phenomenal success in the treatment of depression has unfortunately often overshadowed St John's wort's traditional use as a topical antiseptic and anti-inflammatory wound healer. This salve aims to set the record straight. Great to use on children's cuts and scrapes, and they'll love making the infused oil too, which magically turns from the palest yellow to brilliant scarlet after a couple of weeks on a sunny windowsill.

To make the infused oil:

30–50g St John's wort flowering tops

500ml sunflower oil, to cover

To make the salve:

1 tsp beeswax

50ml infused St John's wort oil

To make the infused oil:

Lightly bruise the flowering tops, then place in a glass jar. Cover with the sunflower oil, then leave to steep on a sunny windowsill, turning occasionally, for up to 1 month. Sunlight is crucial for the reaction to work, and when it has you will be rewarded with an oil that, as if by magic, has turned a bright rusty red colour. If after a month the oil is still clear, leave it a little longer until the sun has done its work – don't worry, it will eventually get there. Once bright red, strain off the spent flowers and discard. The resultant oil can be applied to wounds as it is, or turned into a rich, thick salve perfect to pop into your hand/man-bag.

To make the salve:

In a pan, gently dissolve the beeswax in 50ml infused St John's wort oil on the lowest flame possible – this should take no longer than 1–2 minutes. While still warm, pour into a wide-mouthed jar. The salve will set as it cools.

USE For adults, and children aged 2–16, apply as needed to cover the affected area, up to 3 times a day.

CAUTION Do not expose treated skin to direct sunlight. If any irritation occurs, wash off immediately.

STORAGE The salve will keep in a cool dark place for up to 1 year. The infused oil will keep for 6 months to 1 year.

james's tip When you leave plant material to infuse (especially dried plants), it has a habit of absorbing some of the oil over time. Check every couple of days that all the plant matter is completely covered with oil – just push it back down and add a splash more oil if any is sticking out. That way, you'll extract more of the essential compounds.

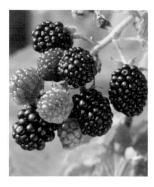

Blackberry Oxymel for Colds

Despite a distinctly modern, almost clinical-sounding name, oxymels are old-fashioned remedies based on a blend of vinegar and honey. They can be used straight or diluted and given as a cordial (as I have done here). With their sticky, sugary flavour, oxymels are a great way to make bitter herbs more palatable as well as an unashamedly underhand way to sneak plant goodness past the lips of children ...

200g blackberries or raspberries

cider or white wine vinegar, to cover

honey, to taste

This is a good one for youngsters suffering from colds – a hot, soothing blackberry drink full of vitamin C; just add honey to taste.

For the cider vinegar, see the recipe on page 31 or use bought.

1 Put the fruit in a clean jar, and cover with the vinegar. Leave for 10 days to 2 weeks, shaking occasionally, then strain through a jelly bag or muslin, mashing the fruit to get the juice out. (You could also rub it through a sieve with the back of a wooden spoon, but make sure you leave all the pips behind.)

2 Pour the liquid into a clean bottle and store in the refrigerator.

USE For adults, and children aged 2–16, this is delicious as a hot drink: put 2–4 teaspoons in a mug, add boiling water and honey to taste.

STORAGE Will keep for up to 1 year in the refrigerator.

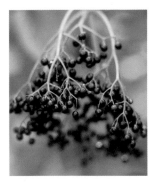

Elderberry Cordial for Colds and Flu

This is a very old recipe, dosed out to countless generations of children (and adults) – a version of it has even been turned into a popular proprietary medicine in the United States. Give a dose at the first sign of colds or flu, especially just before bedtime.

For the juice:

1kg elderberries (or as much as you can pick, preferably on a dry day)

water to cover

To each 600ml juice, add:

450g sugar

12 cloves or 1 cinnamon stick

juice of 1 lime

1 Place the elderberries in a large pan, and just cover with cold water. Stew the fruit for 20 minutes, or until really soft. Strain through muslin, squeezing hard to get out all the juice.

2 Measure the strained elderberry juice into a pan, and for each 600ml juice add 450g sugar, 12 cloves or 1 cinnamon stick, and the juice of 1 lime. Bring slowly to the boil, stirring occasionally to stop the sugar burning, then boil for 15 minutes. Take off the heat and allow to cool.

3 When cold, strain, bottle, and store in the refrigerator.

USE For adults, and children over 6 years: take 1–2 tablespoons in hot water, sipping slowly, up to 3 times a day and especially at bedtime.

STORAGE Will keep for up to 6 months in the refrigerator.

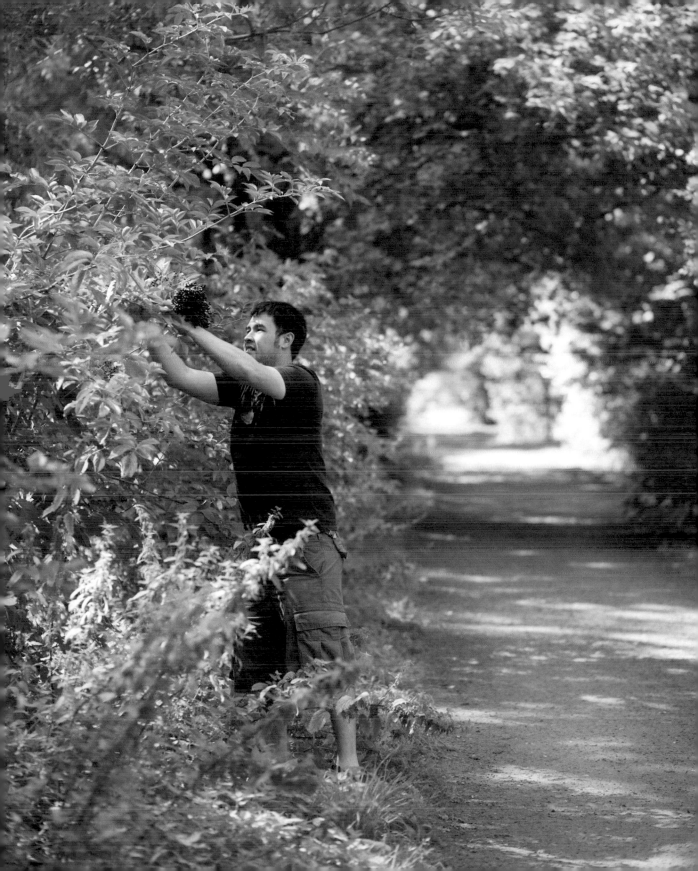

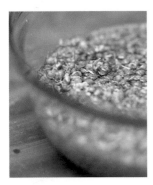

Chamomile and Lavender Massage Rub for Colic

This safe, gentle remedy can help ease the symptoms of colic, using a duo of calming botanical ingredients and the soothing comfort of touch. Chamomile and lavender flowers both contain antispasmodic chemicals that help relieve griping, relax the gut and calm painful spasms.

100g German chamomile (*Matricaria recutita*) flowers, fresh or dried

50g lavender flowers, fresh or dried

400ml olive oil, or to cover

1 Pack the chamomile and lavender flowers loosely in a large jar, and pour the olive oil over to cover all plant material. Seal and leave in a warm place for 2 weeks. Then strain, and bottle.

USE On children over 2, gently massage the oil into the stomach with circular motions, always going clockwise (the same direction as the digestive tract). Also massage into the feet.

STORAGE Store in a cool, dark place for up to 6 months.

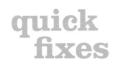

quick fixes

Liquorice Chews for Healthy Teeth

Despite a distinctly unpromising appearance, the intensely sweet flavour of liquorice roots makes them a great sugar-free substitute for more conventional sugary treats. They contain a compound that is up to 50 times sweeter than sugar, making chewing on a stick like gnawing on a solid block of brown sugar. But wait, the best news is yet to come: liquorice not only lacks tooth-rotting sugar but can even go some way towards protecting teeth against cavities by inhibiting bacterial growth and plaque formation. In other words, something sweet and tasty that's actually good for developing teeth! Don't get too carried away with the good news, however: too much liquorice isn't good for you, so limit it to no more than a couple of sticks a week.

Plantain for Nettle Stings

Your grandmother has swindled you. All those years of being told dock was the best thing for nettle stings? Well, it turns out to be not quite true. Plantain, an incredibly common lawn weed, is even better for this purpose. When you're out and about in the countryside and get stung by nettles, crush a few plantain leaves, rub them over the affected area and watch as the redness, pain and tingling subside – in 5–10 minutes.

HOME

Fast, easy, plant-based remedies to help keep your home clean, shiny and sweet-smelling every day of the year.

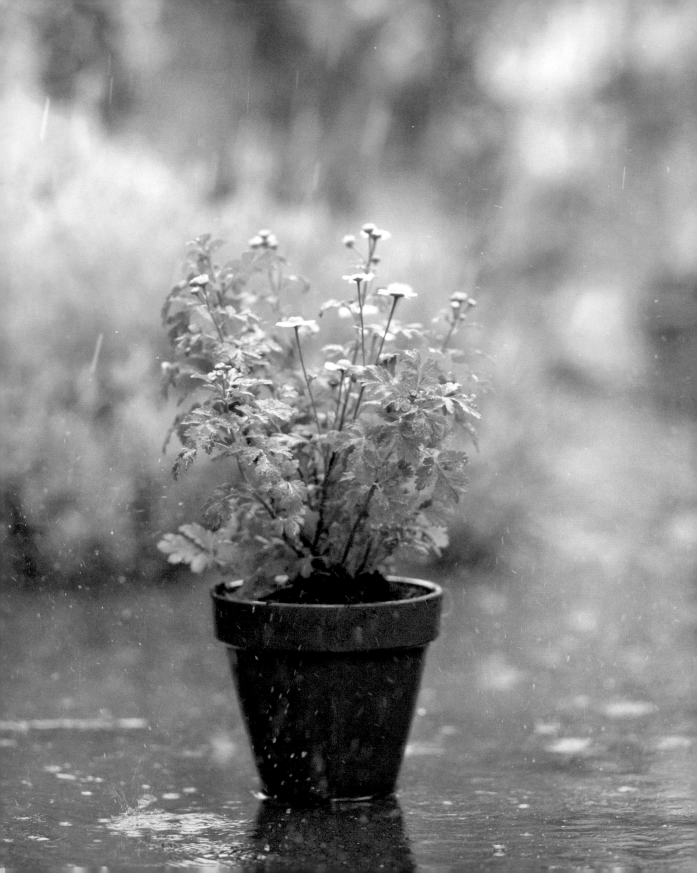

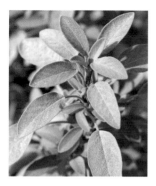

Wormwood and Sage Moth Repellent Sachets

This mix of aromatic herbs will keep those pesky moths from laying the eggs that turn into the larvae which then chomp through your favourite jumpers. These sachets smell lovely to us – but not to the moths. Put a few in cupboards and drawers, alongside the clothes or blankets you want to protect.

2 tbsp dried
  rosemary leaves

2 tbsp dried wormwood
  (*Artemisia
  absinthium*) leaves

2 tbsp dried sage leaves

dash of vodka

1 Strip the leaves from the plants, and crush them finely. Mix together in an open shallow bowl, and sprinkle on a dash of vodka.

2 Put a little of the dried herb mixture into the centre of a small muslin square. Tie with raffia or string. Repeat until you have used up all the herbs.

USE Pop the herbal sachets into cupboards and drawers to deter moths. When they first stop smelling, give them a squeeze and a bash to release more volatile oils. Next time, they will need replacing.

VARIATION SPICY MOTH BAGS
A quick-and-easy moth deterrent: choose a few of the following, whatever you've got on your spice shelf – aniseed, cinnamon bark, caraway seeds, fennel seeds, cardamom pods, cloves, coriander seeds, cumin seeds, peppercorns, dill seeds, celery seeds. Mix your selection together in a bowl. Take a handful of the mix and place in small paper envelopes. Seal and place the envelopes in drawers, wardrobes and clothes chests. The aromatic oils in the spices will be lost over time, so renew occasionally.

An old French recipe for keeping moths at bay: add 2 parts each of dried rosemary, tansy, thyme, mint and southernwood, to 1 part ground cloves. Mix well and put into muslin bags.

'Since I put the mothballs up about 3 weeks ago I haven't seen a single moth – so I think that's an unqualified success.'
Vicky

⚑ gifting These moth sachets make a pretty, practical gift for anyone who cares about keeping their clothes in good nick. Make up a batch of 8 or so bags, arrange them on coloured tissue paper in a pretty gift box, cover with cellophane, tie with a big bow and add a handwritten label.

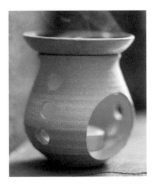

Room Fragrance

Heating essential oils in an oil burner or vaporizer is a quick way to neutralize room odours and create a fragrant, long-lasting aroma. Thyme and eucalyptus are strongly antiseptic, and this scent freshens the air and banishes smells.

3ml lemon essential oil

1ml thyme essential oil

1ml eucalyptus essential oil

❚ Mix the oil together in a brown glass dropper bottle. Shake well.

USE Shake, then put 5 drops in an oil burner/vaporizer and heat gently.

CAUTION Keep away from eyes. Store in a dropper bottle to prevent accidental ingestion.

STORAGE Keeps for 1 year in a brown glass dropper bottle.

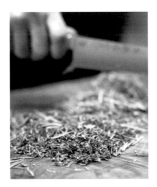

Deodorizer for Sweet-smelling Carpets

To freshen up a stale or grungy carpet, especially after a party, try this simple remedy. The bicarbonate of soda helps neutralize odours and the herbs act as a disinfectant as well as leaving a nice smell on the carpet (and in the vacuum cleaner bag!).

200g bicarbonate of soda

3–4 tbsp dried lavender flowers

3–4 tbsp dried thyme leaves

❚ Mix the bicarbonate of soda, lavender and thyme together in a bowl, then shake over the floor. Leave overnight. Vacuum up the next day.

USE As needed.

STORAGE This makes enough for a normal-sized room but will keep for 1 year in a sealed container.

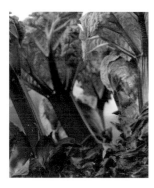

Wood Furniture Polish

Rhubarb root adds a warm golden hue to this natural furniture polish. You can add more rosemary for a stronger scent – or use a different essential oil such as lemon if you prefer. Castile soap is a pure soap available in some supermarkets and pharmacies.

60g rhubarb root (*Rheum rhabarbarum*, *R. rhaponticum* or *R. officinale*)

I litre water

60g beeswax

250ml turpentine

30g grated Castile soap

2 tbsp powdered pine resin

4ml rosemary essential oil

1 First make the rhubarb decoction: put the rhubarb root and water in a pan. Bring to the boil, then simmer for 20–30 minutes. Strain, reserving 500ml of the liquid.

2 Melt the beeswax in a double boiler. Take off the heat and mix in the turpentine; be careful not to be near a naked flame, as the turpentine is flammable.

3 In another double boiler, gently heat 500ml rhubarb decoction with the soap and pine resin until the solids are dissolved.

4 Add the rhubarb mixture to the beeswax and turpentine, and stir. Leave to cool slightly.

5 While cooling, stir in the essential oil. Then pour the polish into a jar and allow to cool completely.

USE Rub a small amount onto the wood using a cloth, then buff with a soft cloth.

STORAGE Will keep for 1–2 years.

Pet Deodorizer

A simple way to keep the bedding of moggies, doggies and other pets coming up smelling of roses – or, at least mint, rosemary and eucalyptus ...

30g dried eucalyptus

30g dried fennel

30g dried mint

30g dried pennyroyal

30g dried rosemary

30g dried wormwood

1 litre water

4 tsp bicarbonate of soda

1ml tea tree essential oil (optional)

1ml thyme essential oil (optional)

1 Place all the dried herbs in a glass bowl and pour over 1 litre freshly boiled water. Cover and leave to steep for 10 minutes. Strain.

2 Dissolve the bicarbonate of soda in the liquid, adding 1ml each of tea tree and thyme essential oils (if you like).

3 Pour the liquid into a spray pump.

USE Once a week, spray on to pet bedding and allow to air dry.

CAUTION If any irritation occurs, consult your vet.

STORAGE Keeps for 2–4 weeks.

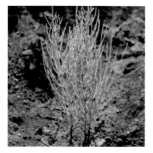

Horsetail Metal Polish

Horsetail – also called pewterwort – has long been used as a metal cleaner because of its high silica content. The tiny crystals act as a mild abrasive to scrub off any dust and grime. There are two ways to apply it: just rub a fresh stem over the metal as a polish or make an infusion and leave the item to soak in it.

50g fresh horsetail stems

1 litre water

To make an infusion, put the chopped horsetail in a pan with the water, and bring to the boil. Leave covered, to cool and infuse overnight.

USE Leave the metal item in the horsetail infusion for 1 hour (or longer if needed). Then wash off and polish with a dry cloth. If using fresh horsetail, rub over well to cover, leave to dry, then buff with a dry cloth.

STORAGE Best used immediately.

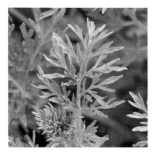

Pet Flea Powder

A traditional mix of herbs used on pets to deter fleas and other insect life. If you use herbs you've gathered yourself, make sure they are properly dried (see page 182). Otherwise, they won't powder finely enough.

4 tbsp dried pennyroyal

2 tbsp dried fennel

2 tbsp dried rosemary

2 tbsp dried wormwood

Put all the herbs together and use a hand blender or a mortar and pestle to grind them to a fine powder.

USE Dust over your dog or cat (avoiding the eyes) once a month. Can also be used to stuff a thin pillow to leave in the pet bed to discourage fleas.

CAUTION If any irritation occurs, consult your vet.

STORAGE Will keep for 1 year in an airtight container.

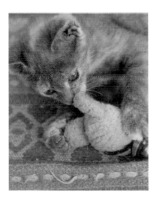

Cat's Christmas Toy

Although everyone knows that cats love catnip, it's less well known that most of them go crazy over valerian too. Apparently, both are used in the big cat enclosures in zoos to keep the lions and tigers entertained. I've mixed the valerian with catnip in this recipe because humans are sometimes less keen on its aromatic smell, but you can make it with 100% catnip if you prefer. This toy will be a much-chased Christmas treat.

small soft toy
or old sock

cat bite-sized pieces
of dried valerian root
(enough to half-fill
your toy)

dried catnip
(to half-fill your toy)

Cut a seam and take the old stuffing out of the soft toy. Fill the toy or old sock with a mixture of dried valerian root and catnip, then sew up to secure. If you are really fond of your cat, you may like to make it a felt mouse, with whiskers and a tail!

STORAGE The dried herbs will last for a few months. If the cat gets tired of the toy, refresh it by restuffing with another batch of valerian and catnip.

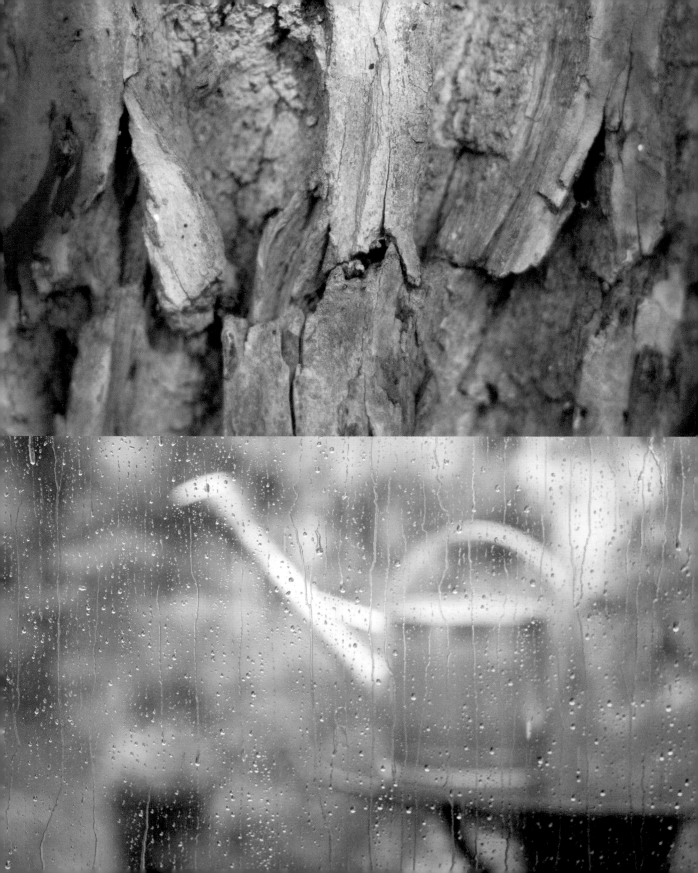

4 THE GROW YOUR OWN DRUGS YEAR

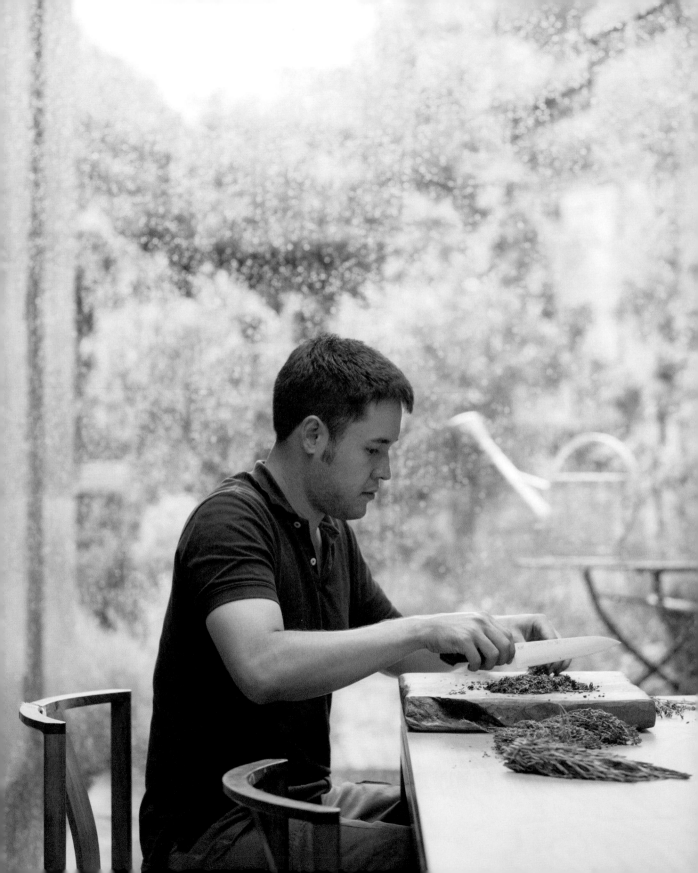

THE SEASONAL GUIDE TO GROWING YOUR OWN PHARMACY

When I was growing up, there were only two seasons: hot and wet and hot and slightly wetter. Sitting on my porch in Singapore, I used to fantasize about the idea of snowball fights, running through autumn leaves and picking spring blossom. I even brought packs of flower bulbs back from summer holidays in the United Kingdom and tried to bring spring to the tropics by putting them in the refrigerator, hoping they might sprout.

Not one of my most successful gardening experiments, I must say, but to an 8-year-old the logic was convincing. Despite my mum's best efforts to convince me that UK weather was not as idyllic as I imagined, I was quite happy to take on a bit of cold and wet in exchange for all the great diversity that seasonal changes bring.

Having now lived here for over 10 years, I must confess that this rose-tinted image has still not lost its gloss, and I am perhaps more passionate than ever about the seasons. As a nation, we are quick to complain about our climate, idealizing warm sunny places, but having lived in one for most of my life I must say they are far less interesting. Yes, you can grow a much wider range of plants in warmer climates and almost everything is in season all year round, but there is not the intense expectation and excitement that seasonal changes bring. To me, nothing can beat the exhilaration of spotting the first snowdrops poking through snow, waiting for just the right time to go bramble-picking and planning the cosy domestic rituals of drying and preserving herbs for the winter months.

Each season brings new ingredients to play with, new challenges to figure out and, of course, new remedies to try, which to me is so much more exciting than doing the same old thing all year round. In this section, I set out my complete seasonal guide to growing, harvesting, drying and storing, showing you exactly what to do when, and giving you my top tips on how to structure the gardening and concocting year. In this way, I hope to help you spot and make use of plants at the peak of their season, even in the darkest depths of winter.

SPRING

sowing and planting

This is the start of the grower's year, a time for planting and digging, sowing and potting. Buy some seeds and watch them grow ... If you're feeling adventurous, propagate some plants from cuttings begged or borrowed from friends and neighbours – no need to buy new ones, you can create and grow your own.

Now is a good time to ...

» Get busy sowing seeds. You don't need a greenhouse: any draught-free indoor windowsill can be used as 'nursery' space if you just want to get your chilli seeds started. Be warned: seed sowing can become extremely addictive; watching those little green shoots rise above the compost is magical.

> **james's tip** If you're planting up a large container with shallow-rooted plants (annuals or Mediterranean-type herbs), break up some old polystyrene packaging and cram a layer at the bottom of the pot, or use upturned plastic flower pots instead. It makes the pot lighter and easier to move around, and you don't need as much compost to fill it.
>
> Don't try this with shrubs, trees or fruit bushes because their roots need the growing room.

» Don't get carried away: if you have only a small garden, patio or pots, you won't need all 100 seeds in the packet to germinate. Sow half this year, then keep the rest dry and dark and they'll be fine for next spring. You'll still end up with plenty of plants for yourself and many more to share or swap.

» To get free plants, why not give propagation a go? Take cuttings of fresh green shoots (with plenty of leaves) from your favourite plants: chamomile, lavender, mints, pelargonium, sage, southernwood, thyme and wormwood all work well. Plant each one in cutting compost nearly up to its leaves, then cover with an upturned plastic bottle, leave it on a warm windowsill and watch it take root.

» Mix and match your planting now, and you'll deter insects throughout the year. Place aromatic plants such as chives, garlic, feverfew, nasturtium, nicotiana, southernwood, tansy, Tagetes (French marigold), thyme, wild marjoram and wormwood near your susceptible roses, fruit and vegetables – many bugs don't like the strong scent they give off. Some of these plants even keep rabbits, hedgehogs and other mammals away ...

» Some plants have thuggish tendencies and will take over your garden given half a chance. Grow invasive plants like bistort, horseradish, horsetail and mint in pots. You can sink their plastic pots into the soil if you like – that way, their roots are contained but they still look as if they're growing in the border.

» As the days lengthen, the soil starts to warm up and light levels rise in mid to late spring. It's all systems go – many seeds can now be planted straight out into the garden – see the spring sowing chart on page 173.

» If you've got a patio or paved area and would like some bouncy greenery underfoot, mix some chamomile or thyme seeds with sand, and pour it into the paving crevices. By summertime, they'll be filled with sweet-smelling plants that release their aroma whenever you walk on them.

» Look out in the wild for ingredients like nettles, plantain, chickweed and dandelion. Their new fresh leafy growth will be perfect for remedy-making now.

» Tidy up your pots. Prune out old growth, give them a water and a feed, and they'll soon be shooting out new leaves.

» Start feeding your potted citrus tree to get it in the best shape for producing strong growth and fruit for your remedies.

» When the risk of frost has passed, move your tender plants outside. Scented-leaved pelargoniums, aloe vera, citrus trees and lemon verbena will be happy soaking up the sun. As will your annuals like basil and nasturtium.

how to plant out
Before you plant any plugs or bought plants out in the garden, give them a drink of water in their pot.

Always dig a bigger hole than you think you'll need: it's easier for new roots to find their way into soil already broken up with a spade or trowel. Add a couple of handfuls of grit or sand to the hole and mix in. Take the plant from the pot and place in the hole so the soil is at the same level as it was in the pot. This stops the stems rotting. Backfill with soil, firm well with your hands or a careful foot, and water in well.

growing berries
Many recipes for children (and the respiratory system, too) make use of berries, especially bilberries, blackberries, blackcurrants, cranberries, elderberries and raspberries.

Berries grow on canes or bushes and are easy to cultivate in the garden – or find elderberries and blackberries in the wild. Plant them in winter or early spring. They can even be grown in pots if you're short of space. Here's how:

Cane Fruit (blackberries and raspberries)
You can buy bundles of cane blackberry (*Rubus fruticosus*) and raspberry (*Rubus idaeus*) cheaply in autumn and winter from garden centres or nurseries. They come 'bare-root', tied together in bundles of 5 or 10. Don't be alarmed by the sight of these seemingly dead sticks, they're dormant but will start growing when it warms up. You can also buy cane fruit in pots from garden centres in spring. Before planting, soak bare-root canes in a bucket of water overnight. Add some organic matter to the planting hole, then place the plants about 1 metre apart. Firm well in and water.

Cane fruit needs support to grow well. Stretch a few strands of wire horizontally between two posts – you can then tie in the canes to the wire as they grow. If you have space for only a couple of plants, keep them in check with a wigwam of bamboo canes. As the fruits swell in the spring and early summer, it is important to keep them well watered, especially during sunny spells.

Bush Fruit (bilberries, blackcurrants, cranberries)

Again look out for bare-root plants in winter and containerized plants in the spring. They're reasonably priced and surprisingly high-yielding even from the first year. Blackcurrants (*Ribes nigrum*) will tolerate a little shade, but like rich, moisture-retentive soil. Bilberries (*Vaccinium myrtillus*) and cranberries (*Vaccinium macrocarpon*) produce great fruit and fabulous autumn leaf colour. They need a sheltered spot and acid soil; you can buy acid-high ericaceous compost from garden centres. They flower in spring, with the fruit developing through the summer months. They produce a good crop on a single plant, but for optimum yield try growing a couple of different varieties together. Keep very well watered, using rainwater whenever you can; install a water butt or keep out a bucket to collect rainfall.

Berries in Pots

It is possible to grow cane and bush fruit in pots. You'll need a large pot with a crock (a piece of broken terracotta) over the holes in the bottom for drainage, and a good, peat-free compost enriched generously with well-rotted manure or garden compost. Remember that the plants will have access only to the nutrients you give them, so regular feeding and watering is important. Cane fruit will need support for their tall, flexible stems. If they're grown against a wall, you can tie them in to horizontal wires or a piece of trellis. Otherwise place a wigwam of bamboo canes in the pot.

a mixed pot to raise your spirits

To help lift your mood when you're feeling low, plant up a mixed pot with lemon balm, rose root, St John's wort and vervain – all are used to soothe anxiety and nervous tension. Buy small new plants from a nursery or garden centre and by mid-summer you'll be reaping the harvest ...

In a 50cm diameter pot, place a crock (or a couple of flat stones) over the drainage holes in the bottom. Three-quarters fill the pot with peat-free compost, thoroughly mixing in a handful of pelleted chicken manure (any fertilizer in direct contact with a plant's roots can burn them). Have a go at arranging your plants in the pot: lemon balm grows tall and will make a great centrepiece, vervain and rose root will trail over the edges and soften the look, St John's wort will provide a sunny little filler. Then plant them in: turn each well-watered herb upside down, give it a gentle squeeze and tap it out into your hand. Place each plant in its spot, fill around with more compost, firm well and water. The compost should settle to about 2–3cm below the top of the pot – you don't want it full to the brim as you'll need space to water.

Water each day in dry periods. Even when it has rained, check how moist the container is; many pot plants can drink a surprising amount. A foliar feed every so often will do it a world of good too – use some of your home-made comfrey or nettle tonic (see page 176). Then simply harvest the leaves and flowering tops to make teas and tinctures as you need them.

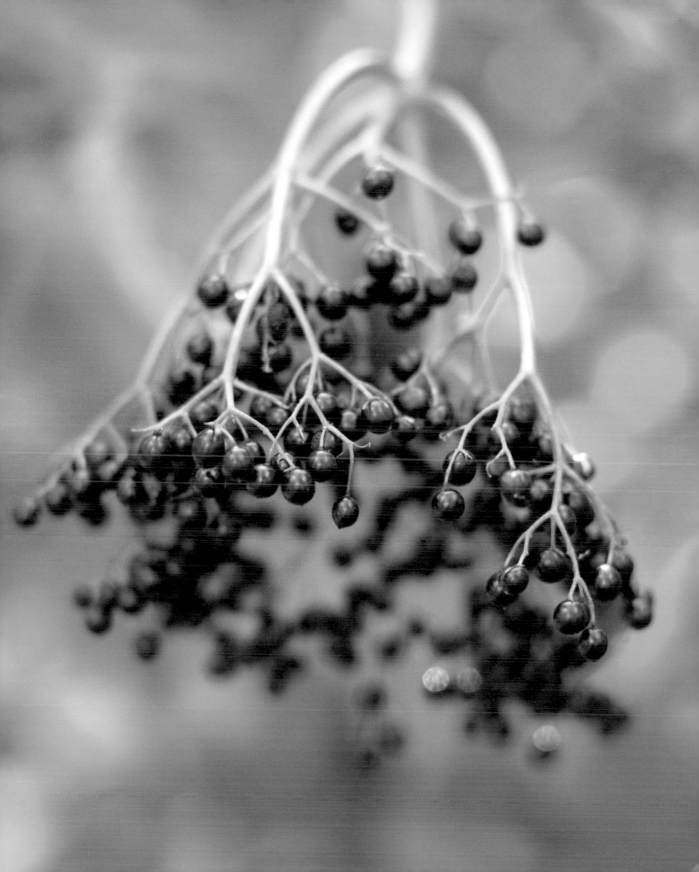

plant a chamomile seat

If you've got an old stone seat, wooden bench or even a low wall in your garden, you can make a chamomile seat to relax on.

Use the bouncy, low-growing, non-flowering chamomile 'Treneague': it's very fragrant, lush and otherworldly; you'll feel as if you're sitting at the bottom of the sea!

1   The first step is to make sure that the surface of your new seat is solid and weight-bearing. It can be any material, from concrete to brickwork and even wood (as long as it has been treated with a good wood preservative). We used a rectangle of wood with a very small lip round the edges (not too high, or it would cut into your legs), which we dropped into a brick wall almost like the fabric seat of a chair dropping into its frame.

2   To ensure good drainage, so the plant roots are not sitting in water for long periods of time, spread a layer of gravel over the base, about 2–3cm deep.

3   Spread a layer of soil or loam-based compost on top of the gravel, about 3–5cm deep.

4   You can buy chamomile as turf (in 1m squares; see Stockists, page 215) or in trays of small thumb-sized plugs, which works out cheaper. The plugs are also great for planting in any crevices you have in your paving, releasing their aroma as you walk over them. Lay the turf or plant the plugs about 15cm apart.

5   Site your seat in a sunny area, water well and allow to establish, watching out for weeds. It won't take constant, heavy wear but it will provide you with a beautifully scented garden feature. Once established, there's very little maintenance – perhaps an occasional trim with garden shears.

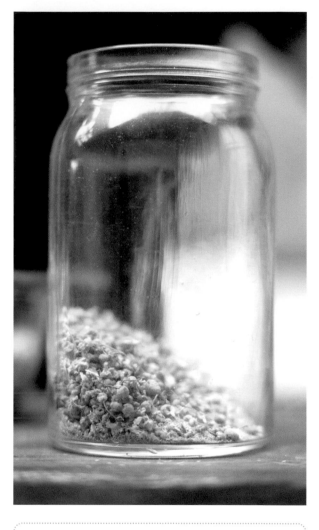

james's tip People often set beer traps for slugs and snails (jam jars sunk in the ground half-full of beer; anything that slithers in meets a watery grave). Upturned grapefruit skins work just as well, though. Eat your grapefruit for breakfast, then place the empty halves on the ground at night. When you go out in the early morning, you'll find the slugs have congregated for easy disposal and your young seedlings are safe.

SPRING: SOWING CHART

In early spring, you can start sowing many of the plants below in seed trays, keeping them indoors to germinate. The rest can be scattered in late spring directly into the garden (or in pots) wherever you want them to grow. Sow them outdoors in shallow drills, lightly cover with compost or soil, and water. Once the seedlings grow, thin them out a bit to leave the strongest ones to produce healthy plants.

✱ *The potential health benefits of the plants listed below are based on their traditional use.*

Black mustard *Brassica nigra*, seeds applied topically to encourage circulation and soothe muscle pain. Sow outdoors.

Caraway *Carum carvi*, seeds used to aid digestion. Sow outdoors.

Chamomile *Matricaria recutita*, used for indigestion, skin irritations, as a mild sedative for anxiety, and to lighten blonde hair. Sow in seed trays to germinate.

Chilli *Capsicum* spp., stimulant, pain reliever used topically for muscular aches and pains, to encourage circulation, can also help thin phlegm in stubborn coughs. Grow in pots, germinate indoors.

Coriander *Coriandrum sativum*, to aid digestion and soothe stomachs. Sow outdoors.

Cornflower *Centaurea cyanus*, traditionally used for soothing and brightening eyes, and cosmetically as hair rinse. Sow outdoors once frosts have passed.

Dill *Anethum graveolens*, traditionally used for digestion, gas and intestinal spasms. Sow outdoors.

Echinacea *Echinacea angustifolia, E. purpurea* or *E. pallida*; helps stimulate the immune system and lessen the severity and duration of cold and flu symptoms. Plant in seed trays first to germinate.

Fennel *Foeniculum vulgare*, to help ease bloating and stomach upsets, applied topically as an eyewash. Sow outdoors.

Feverfew *Tanacetum parthenium*, preventative treatment for migraine, and can be helpful with fever. Plant in plug modules first to germinate. Will self-seed prolifically once established. DO NOT USE IF PREGNANT OR BREASTFEEDING, UNDER 18, OR HAVE A STOMACH OR MOUTH ULCER.

Flax *Linum usitatissimum*, the seeds (known as linseed) used as a laxative, for coughs and bronchitis, topically for burns, and as a phytoestrogen. Sow outdoors.

Goji berries *Lycium barbarum*, can help stimulate the immune system in colds and flu. Sow outdoors or buy in a pot.

Goldenrod *Solidago virgaurea*, antiseptic used as tea to soothe urinary tract infections and kidney stones. Sow in seed trays to germinate.

Hollyhock *Alcea rosea*, soothing for sore throats. Sow outdoors.

Lemon balm *Melissa officinalis*, calming, helps soothe nervous tension and relieve anxiety. Applied topically to treat cold sores. Sow outdoors.

Marigold *Calendula officinalis*, soothes rashes, bites and burns and can speed skin healing, also used as a stomach soother. Sow outdoors.

Nasturtium *Tropaeolum majus*, used as a mild diuretic and decongestant for catarrh and upper respiratory tract infections. Peppery leaves and flowers used in salads. Sow outdoors later in the season.

Onion *Allium cepa*, antiseptic, anti-inflammatory; good all-round health tonic, encourages production of phlegm. Plant as sets (small immature bulbs) in early spring.

Pansy *Viola tricolor*, used topically for eczema, acne and skin disorders; anti-inflammatory and gentle diuretic, and can loosen chest congestion. Sow outdoors.

Parsley *Petroselinum crispum*, diuretic, used for digestive problems and anaemia. DO NOT USE IF YOU HAVE KIDNEY PROBLEMS. Sow outdoors.

Pennyroyal *Mentha pulegium*, used as an insect repellent. DO NOT USE INTERNALLY. Sow in plug modules first to germinate, then plant outside in early summer.

Rocket *Eruca vesicaria* subsp. *sativa*, flavoursome, peppery leaves used in salads. Sow outdoors.

Sage *Salvia officinalis*, helps loosen mucus in the upper respiratory tract, soothe the throat; used for hot flushes and sweating during menopause. Sow in seed trays to germinate, or buy as a small plant.

St John's wort *Hypericum perforatum*, can ease mild to moderate depression, anxiety and Seasonal Affective Disorder (SAD), used topically as a wound healer. Sow in seed trays to germinate.

Tansy *Tanacetum vulgare*, insect repellent. Sow outdoors.

Vervain *Verbena officinalis*, gentle mood-improver and nerve-soother, can aid indigestion. Sow outdoors.

Wild lettuce *Lactuca virosa*, mild sedative used to ease insomnia and stress. Sow outdoors.

Wild strawberry *Fragaria vesca*, both leaves and fruit are mildly astringent and diuretic and used cosmetically in face packs. Sow outdoors.

Wormwood *Artemisia absinthium*, a digestive 'bitter' to ease bloating and increase appetite in small doses, insect repellent. Sow in seed trays to germinate or buy as a small plant.

SPRING: FRESH LEAVES FOR PICKING

If you've got the plants below growing indoors or out, you can pick leaves now on a cut-and-come-again basis – astonishingly, the more you pick, the more grow (within reason of course!).

* *The potential health benefits of the plants listed below are based on their traditional use.*

Aloe vera *Aloe barbadensis*, the gel soothes burns and skin problems, speeds healing time of cuts and wounds.

Angelica *Angelica archangelica*, anti-inflammatory, can help relieve flatulence and indigestion, and loosen respiratory catarrh. Stems can be candied for cooking.

Bay *Laurus nobilis*, aids digestion, used in aftershaves and colognes for its pungent aroma.

Eucalyptus *Eucalyptus* spp., decongestant for colds and coughs, antiseptic in sore throat and skin treatments, good insect repellent.

Fennel *Foeniculum vulgare*, to help ease bloating and stomach upsets, applied topically as an eyewash.

Lemon balm *Melissa officinalis*, calming, helps soothe nervous tension and relieve anxiety. Applied topically to treat cold sores.

Lemongrass *Cymbopogon citratus*, aids digestion, antibiotic, and insect repellent.

Mint *Mentha* spp., often used to help with bloating, dyspepsia and irritable bowel syndrome, applied topically as an antiseptic and to soothe itching.

Nettle *Urtica dioica*, highly nutritious tonic, may help with hay fever, used as an anti-dandruff rinse for hair and to improve shine.

Parsley *Petroselinum crispum*, diuretic, used for digestive problems and anaemia. DO NOT USE IF YOU HAVE KIDNEY PROBLEMS.

Rosemary *Rosmarinus officinalis*, reputed to help memory and concentration, and increase alertness. Applied topically for muscle pain.

Sage *Salvia officinalis*, helps loosen mucus in the upper respiratory tract, soothe the throat, used for hot flushes and sweating during menopause. Harvest leaves just before flowers bloom.

Tarragon *Artemisia dracunculus*, aromatic herb used in aftershaves and colognes.

Thyme *Thymus vulgaris* or wild thyme (*Thymus serpyllum*), antiseptic, especially for the mouth, used to help loosen phlegm, applied topically to ease rheumatic pains, insecticidal.

Wild marjoram *Origanum vulgare*, antiseptic used to soothe respiratory tract and urinary infections.

Willow bark *Salix* spp., for pain relief, especially in rheumatic disorders and headaches. DO NOT GIVE TO UNDER-18s OR ANYONE ALLERGIC TO ASPIRIN.

SUMMER

weeding and watering

This is the most exciting time of the year, when everything in the garden is at full tilt. Borders and pots are cascading with leafy growth and flowers are ready to harvest. You need to watch the watering – containers can dry out surprisingly quickly at this time of year – and keep up with the weeding. But mainly this is when you'll start enjoying the richness of the garden and reaping the medicinal and culinary harvest of growing your own.

Now is a good time to ...

» If you haven't already done so, sow seeds of annuals like basil, cornflower and pot marigold now. They'll quickly germinate and are useful fillers – you can pop them into any spaces in your borders, pots or window boxes.

» Keep on top of watering (and feeding), particularly where containers are concerned – you might find you're doing a daily round with the watering can.

» Start making comfrey and nettle foliar (leaf) feeds for the garden. Find a big bucket, then fill it with nettles, feverfew or comfrey leaves. Pour water over, cover, and leave for 2 weeks or more until it's nice and smelly. Decant into a watering can or large spray bottle. Give the leaves of outdoor plants a good soaking, either in the early morning or late evening (to stop the sun from scorching them).

» Enjoy harvesting from mid-summer onwards. Use plants fresh. But if you've a glut of any ingredients, dry them for use at a later date. This is particularly good for rose petals, bunches of herbs and some chillies. Chillies can also be stored in oil.

» After they've flowered, you can give a gentle deadhead to echinacea, elecampane, lavender, lemon verbena, marshmallow, mint, pot marigold, sage, tansy, thyme, vervain and wild marjoram to promote new growth. Also trim feverfew, lady's mantle, lemon balm, St John's wort and yarrow to prevent rampant self-seeding.

grow speedy watercress

Watercress (*Nasturtium officinale*) is a vitamin- and mineral-rich general health tonic that is easy to grow:

Put some clean pebbles in a bowl, then half-fill with mineral-rich spring water. Use a bunch of supermarket watercress, but try to get the best quality, as it can be a bit limp. Poke some holes in the pebbles and stick in the watercress cuttings, so they stand upright. It will quickly send out its own roots and you'll soon have fresh watercress.

After about 6 weeks, you'll need to clean out the bowl and start again. Just make up another bowlful using your leftover watercress and off you go...

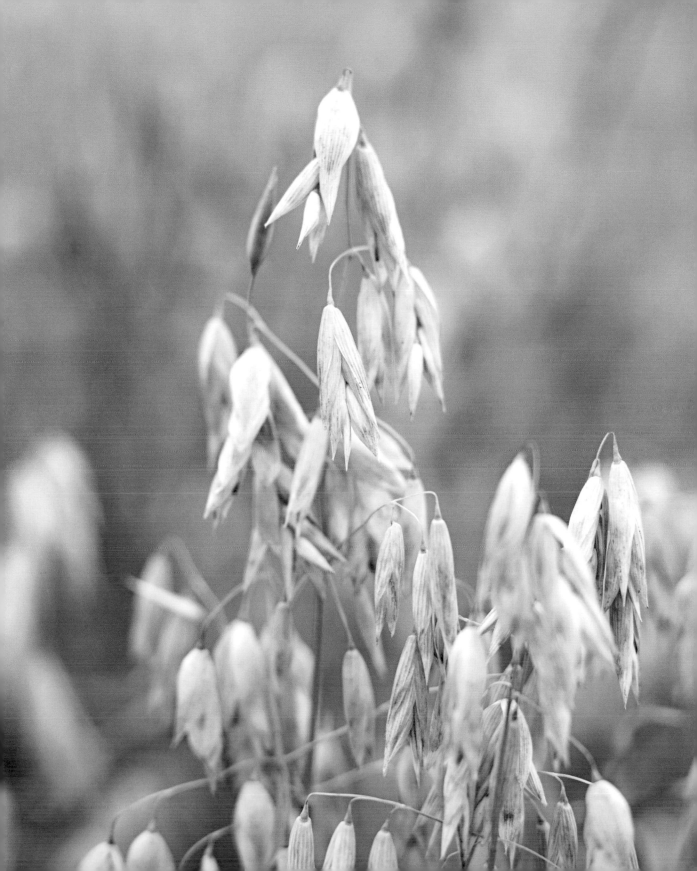

SUMMER: PICKINGS FROM THE WILD

The plants below are easy to find now in hedgerows, meadows, woodland, wasteland and other wild places. Before you pick them, read our foraging guidelines on page 208.

* *The potential health benefits of the plants listed below are based on their traditional use.*

Blackberry *Rubus fruticosus*, fruits are high in vitamin C, both leaves and fruit are mildly astringent and are used to treat diarrhoea.

Chickweed *Stellaria media*, anti-inflammatory and mild diuretic, applied topically to soothe itchy skin, and packed with vitamins – eat as a salad green.

Dandelion *Taraxacum officinale*, general diuretic, health tonic, anti-inflammatory. The young leaves are good in teas and salads, the flowers applied topically in oil and creams for sore muscles and arthritis.

Elder *Sambucus nigra*, has antiviral properties and helps speed recovery from colds and flu, anti-inflammatory. Can use leaves, flowers and berries, BUT DO NOT EAT THE BERRIES RAW.

Eyebright *Euphrasia* spp., helps soothe inflamed tissues around the eyes, and is traditionally used to treat conjunctivitis. Harvest the leaves and flowers. Semi-parasitic plant that is unsuitable for growing in gardens.

Hawthorn *Crataegus monogyna* or *C. laevigata*, tonic for heart health and circulatory diseases. Harvest the leaves, flowers and berries.

Herb Robert *Geranium robertianum*, applied topically can help soothe skin conditions and inflammation. Harvest the leaves.

Horsetail *Equisetum arvense*, traditionally used for cystitis and to help improve thin, brittle hair and nails. Harvest the leaves.

Ivy *Hedera helix*, used in cosmetic treatments to help cellulite. The leaves are used in expectorant cough mixtures. DO NOT EAT THE BERRIES. Harvest the leaves.

Meadowsweet *Filipendula ulmaria*, anti-inflammatory, soothes acid stomachs, analgesic. DO NOT GIVE TO UNDER-16s OR ANYONE ALLERGIC TO ASPIRIN. Pick the flowering tops – it thrives in wet ditches and marshy meadows.

Nettle *Urtica dioica*, highly nutritious tonic, may help with hay fever, used as an anti-dandruff rinse for hair and to improve shine. Harvest the young leaves and flowering tops.

Plantain *Plantago lanceolata*, mild diuretic, anti-inflammatory, antihistamine, soothes nettle stings, and helps stem bleeding and heal wounds. Harvest the leaves.

Spruce *Picea* spp., apply topically for skin disorders; decongestant inhalation. Harvest the needles.

> **james's tip** Mulch isn't just for the borders; it can work wonders on your pots and containers too. You can really go to town on this, using ornamental gravel, coloured glass chips, recycled rubber chips, anything that suits your style. A mulch will stop weeds, keep water in and deter pests, as slugs and snails won't like crawling over sharp gravel or grit to get to their lunch.

SUMMER: FRESH LEAVES FOR PICKING

The leaves of the plants below are ready to be picked now and throughout the growing season. Go for fresh new growth – it'll contain more active ingredients and taste better too.

✱ *The potential health benefits of the plants listed below are based on their traditional use.*

Agrimony *Agrimonia eupatoria*, a 'bitter' for stomach problems including diarrhoea and colitis; mild diuretic.

Aloe vera *Aloe barbadensis*, soothes burns and skin problems, speeds healing time of cuts and wounds.

Basil *Ocimum basilicum*, antibacterial, but mostly used as a fragrant aromatic in aftershaves and colognes.

Bay *Laurus nobilis*, aids digestion, used in aftershaves and colognes for its pungent aroma.

Coriander *Coriandrum sativum*, to aid digestion and soothe the stomach.

Dill *Anethum graveolens*, traditionally used for digestion, gas and intestinal spasms. Use leaves in salads and cooking.

Eucalyptus *Eucalyptus* spp., decongestant for colds and coughs, antiseptic in sore throats and skin treatments, good insect repellent.

Feverfew *Tanacetum parthenium*, preventative treatment for migraine, and can be helpful in fever. DO NOT USE IF PREGNANT OR BREASTFEEDING, UNDER 18, OR HAVE A STOMACH OR MOUTH ULCER.

Gotu kola *Centella asiatica*, to soothe skin conditions, aid wound healing, and for aching joints and muscles.

Greater celandine *Chelidonium majus*, traditionally used for gall-bladder conditions and applied topically for warts, corns and eczema.

Lady's mantle *Alchemilla mollis*, traditionally used to help stem bleeding, lighten menstrual flow and for diarrhoea.

Lemon balm *Melissa officinalis*, calming, helps soothe nervous tension and relieve anxiety. Applied topically to treat cold sores.

Lemongrass *Cymbopogon citratus*, insect repellent and antifungal agent.

Marshmallow *Althaea officinalis*, contains mucilage to soothe gastrointestinal tract, coughs and sore throats, soothing and softening for skin.

Mint *Mentha* spp., often used to help with bloating, dyspepsia and irritable bowel syndrome, applied topically as an antiseptic and to soothe itching.

Olive *Olea europaea*, oil used as an emollient for skin and in cooking, leaves used for mildly elevated blood pressure and to help control blood sugar levels.

james's tip Tie in your climbers, but don't splash out on expensive tree ties; a pair of old tights is all you need. Cut the legs into strips about 2.5cm wide so that you end up with a number of 'hoops', then snip these into elastic lengths of material that can be used for tying plants to their supports. The tights will become invisible in no time and are good and stretchy so they won't damage the plants.

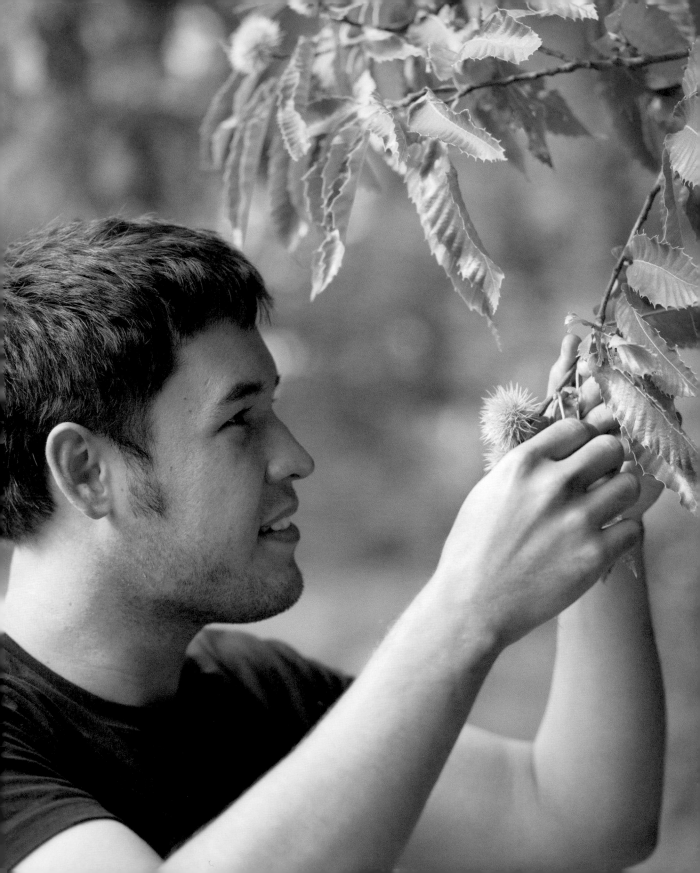

Parsley *Petroselinum crispum*, diuretic, used for digestive problems and anaemia. DO NOT USE IF YOU HAVE KIDNEY PROBLEMS.

Pelargonium *Pelargonium* spp., the scented-leaved varieties are used in skin treatments, cosmetics and pot-pourri.

Pennyroyal *Mentha pulegium*, used as an insect repellent. DO NOT USE INTERNALLY.

Raspberry *Rubus idaeus*, leaves traditionally used to aid childbirth, can help with menopausual symptoms and diarrhoea, and can be used as an eye lotion and mouthwash.

Rocket *Eruca vesicaria* subsp. *sativa*, flavoursome, peppery leaves used in salads.

Rosemary *Rosmarinus officinalis*, reputed to help memory and concentration and increase alertness. Applied topically for muscle pain.

Sage *Salvia officinalis*, helps loosen mucus in the upper respiratory tract, soothes the throat; and used for hot flushes and sweating during menopause. Harvest leaves just before flowers bloom.

Skullcap *Scutellaria lateriflora*, used to help soothe nervous agitation.

Southernwood *Artemisia abrotanum*, for digestive and liver problems, insect repellent.

Tansy *Tanacetum vulgare*, insect repellent.

Tarragon *Artemisia dracunculus*, aromatic herb used in aftershaves and colognes.

Tea *Camellia sinensis*, antioxidant, antibacterial, astringent, gentle stimulant due to the caffeine content.

Thyme *Thymus vulgaris* or wild thyme (*Thymus serpyllum*), antiseptic, especially for the mouth, used to help loosen phlegm, applied topically to ease rheumatic pains, insecticidal.

Vervain *Verbena officinalis*, gentle mood-improver and nerve-soother, can aid indigestion.

Wild lettuce *Lactuca virosa*, mild sedative to ease insomnia and stress.

Wild marjoram *Origanum vulgare*, antiseptic used to soothe respiratory and urinary tract infections.

Witch hazel *Hamamelis virginiana*, used as an anti-inflammatory and to stem bleeding, leaves and twigs are used to soothe bruises, sprains and skin conditions.

Wormwood *Artemisia absinthium*, a digestive 'bitter' to ease bloating and increase appetite in small doses, insect repellent.

james's tip If you're going away for a few days and want to keep your plants watered, group them together on the kitchen draining board, sitting on one end of an old bath towel. Put the other end of the towel in the sink full of water. The towel will act like a wick and keep your plants alive.

drying leaves

Pick leaves for drying on a sunny day, about mid-morning, as by then the dew has evaporated and the essential oils are at their peak.

Leaves are generally at their best just before the plant flowers – choose fresh, green ones, avoiding any that are discoloured or diseased. You can cut whole stems of short-leaved herbs such as thyme or wild marjoram; but pick larger leaves, such as basil or lady's mantle, individually. Don't go overboard – you won't need masses of them (dried leaves last for only 1 year).

First make sure the leaves are clean and free of insects; don't wash them, just give them a quick wipe if needed. Place them on slatted wooden trays or wire trays covered with muslin; air needs to circulate beneath and around them. Then leave in a warm, dark, well-ventilated space – an airing cupboard or warm loft space is ideal. You're aiming for a temperature of about 20–32°C (68–90°F). Check every couple of days, until the leaves are dry and papery – it might take up to 1 week. Once dried, you can strip them off their stems and crumble them, or store them whole. Keep in an airtight glass jar or container in a dry, dark place for up to 1 year. Dried leaves are about twice as strong as fresh, so use half the quantities if substituting for fresh in the recipes.

quick drying method

If you need dried leaves quickly, try oven-drying. Space the leaves well apart on a baking tray covered with greaseproof paper, then place in the oven on the lowest setting, with the door open. Leave for a couple of hours, checking regularly – you want the leaves to be papery but not so crispy they crumble into dust. Once ready, use at once or store in an airtight container as above.

SUMMER: FRESH FLOWERS FOR PICKING

Flowers are best harvested just as they come into bloom – you can use them fresh in remedies now or dry them to use during winter. Here are a few to look out for.

* *The potential health benefits of the plants listed below are based on their traditional use.*

Agrimony *Agrimonia eupatoria*, a 'bitter' for stomach problems including diarrhoea and colitis, mild diuretic.

Chamomile *Matricaria recutita*, for indigestion, skin irritations, mild sedative for anxiety, and to lighten blonde hair.

Cornflower *Centaurea cyanus*, traditionally used for soothing and brightening eyes, and cosmetically as a hair rinse.

Echinacea *Echinacea angustifolia*, *E. purpurea* or *E. pallida*, helps stimulate the immune system and lessen the severity and duration of cold and flu symptoms.

Elderflower *Sambucus nigra*, has antiviral properties and helps speed recovery from colds and flu, anti–inflammatory, delicious made into cordials.

Goldenrod *Solidago virgaurea*, antiseptic used as tea to soothe urinary tract infections and kidney stones. Pick flowering tops and leaves.

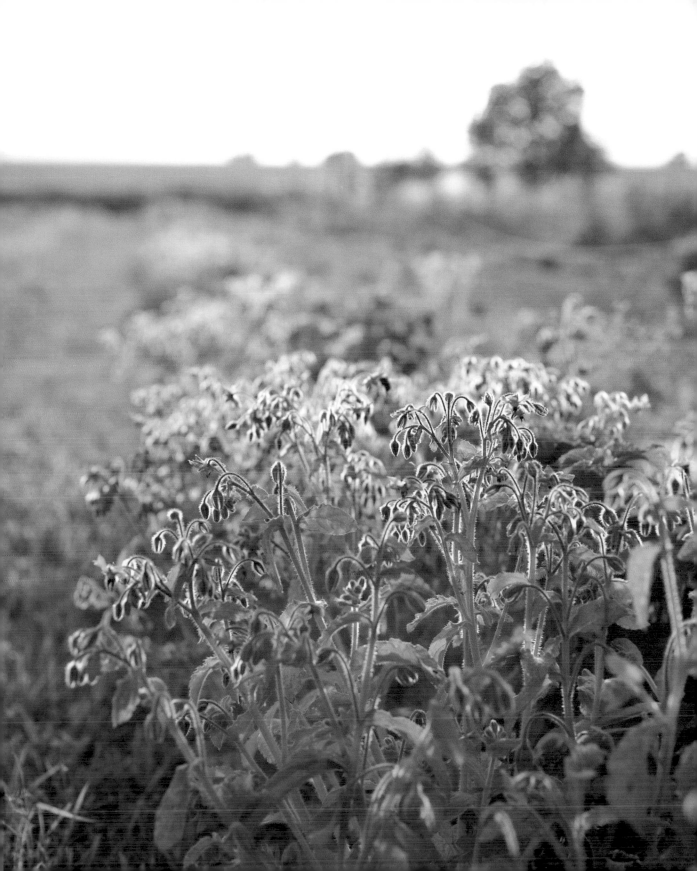

Hollyhock *Alcea rosea*, soothing for sore throats and coughs.

Honeysuckle *Lonicera japonica*, anti-inflammatory and antiseptic, gentle painkiller used for sore throats and headaches.

Jasmine *Jasminum grandiflorum*, anti-inflammatory, soothing for sore throats.

Lavender *Lavandula angustifolia*, soothing, can help ease nervous tension, antiseptic, wound healing.

Lime (linden) flowers *Tilia* spp., traditionally used for fevers and to calm anxiety.

Marigold *Calendula officinalis*, soothes rashes, bites and burns and can speed skin healing, stomach soother.

Mullein *Verbascum thapsus*, expectorant and decongestant, mild analgesic used for earache.

Nasturtium *Tropaeolum majus*, used as a mild diuretic and decongestant for catarrh and upper respiratory tract infections. Peppery leaves and flowers used in salads.

Pansy *Viola tricolor*, used topically for eczema, acne and skin disorders, anti-inflammatory and gentle diuretic, and can loosen chest congestion.

Rose *Rosa gallica*, *R. damascena* and other cultivars used for flavouring and scent, and as a mild stress-reliever.

Skullcap *Scutellaria lateriflora*, used to help soothe nervous agitation.

St John's wort *Hypericum perforatum*, can ease mild to moderate depression, anxiety and SAD, used topically as a wound healer.

Vervain *Verbena officinalis*, gentle mood-improver and nerve-soother, can aid indigestion.

Wormwood *Artemisia absinthium*, a digestive 'bitter' to ease bloating and increase appetite in small doses, insect repellent.

Yarrow *Achillea millefolium*, traditionally used for nosebleeds and wounds to improve healing, and to aid digestion. Use leaves and flowering tops.

drying flowers

Harvest flowers for drying when the buds have just opened.

Aim to pick them on a sunny mid-morning, after the dew has evaporated. (If the flowers are damp, mould can set in.) Wipe them gently with a dry cloth to clean, if needed, and remove any insects. You can harvest them as single blooms (chamomile, pot marigold); as flowering tops (St John's wort, nettles); as petals (roses); or as flowerheads (elderflower, yarrow). Long-stalked, small flowers such as lavender are best dried by hanging upside down in bunches from the stalks, with a paper bag tied over the flowerheads.

To air-dry flowers, place them on slatted wooden trays or wire trays covered with muslin – you want air to circulate around them. Place in a warm, dark, well-ventilated and dry place – an airing cupboard or warm loft space is ideal. You want a temperature of about 20–32°C (68–90°F). Leave for a few days, checking occasionally to see if they are dry and papery – the process might take up to a week. Once dried, you can store the flowers whole or as petals, or crumble them, depending on how you want to use them. Store in an airtight glass jar or container in a dry, dark place. Dried flowers will keep for up to 1 year.

SUMMER: FRESH FRUIT AND VEGETABLES FOR PICKING

Pick fruit and vegetables just as they are starting to get ripe – you can use them fresh in remedies at once, infuse them in oils or freeze them for use during the winter months. Here are some to look out for.

✳ *The potential health benefits of the plants listed below are based on their traditional use.*

Bilberry *Vaccinium myrtillus*, rich in vitamin C and anthocyanosides, often used for eye health and vascular conditions such as varicose veins and piles.
Blackcurrant *Ribes nigrum*, rich in vitamin C and anthocyanosides, may help in maintaining cardiovascular health.
Chilli *Capsicum* spp., stimulant, pain reliever used topically for muscular aches and pains, to encourage circulation, can also help thin phlegm in stubborn coughs.
Cranberry *Vaccinium macrocarpon*, for treatment and prevention of mild urinary tract infections.
Garlic *Allium sativum*, all-rounder for colds, flu, helps lower cholesterol, antifungal. Lift bulbs and leave to dry for a few days in the sun before using.
Lemon *Citrus limon*, antibacterial and astringent on skin, high in vitamin C.

Lime *Citrus aurantifolia*, antibacterial and astringent on skin, high in vitamin C.
Onion *Allium cepa*, encourages production of phlegm, antiseptic, anti-inflammatory. Good all-round health tonic. Lift bulbs and leave to dry for a few days in the sun before using.
Orange *Citrus aurantium*, contains vitamin C, rind used to ease digestive pain.
Peach *Prunus persica*, delicious fruit.
Raspberry *Rubus idaeus*, high in vitamin C, used in children's cordials.
Watercress *Nasturtium officinale*, vitamin and mineral-rich, general health tonic.
Wild strawberry *Fragaria vesca*, mild astringent, used cosmetically in face packs, etc.

freezing fruits

Many summer fruits freeze very well, especially soft fruits such as bilberries, blackberries, blackcurrants, cherries, plums and raspberries.

Pick them on a dry day, handling them carefully so as not to bruise them. Remove any stalks or stones. Place the fruits individually on plastic freezing trays, then freeze for a few hours. Once frozen, you can pack them together into large freezer bags or cartons, then label and date. They'll last for 6 months or so. Strawberries are the exception: they don't like freezing, but you can puree and then freeze them, or make them into delicious jams instead.

freezing herbs

In late summer, you can freeze fresh basil, lemongrass, mint and other culinary herbs. Pick the leaves and put them straight on to a flat layer of silver foil, then fold a layer of silver foil over. Label with the date and then freeze. Use frozen leaves in recipes and remedies as you would fresh ones.

AUTUMN

berry and root harvesting

In autumn, most plants are starting to shut up shop and prepare for their dormant season. The blooms are going, going, gone, leaves are beginning to fall, but there are still fruits and roots to be harvested and seeds to be collected, ready to kickstart next year's growth.

Now is the time to ...

» Plant your garlic sets (small immature bulbs) out in the garden, as they need a cold spell to thrive. Leave just the small tips protruding from the soil.

» Collect seeds (see list below), and store them in paper bags or envelopes for sowing next year or for use in remedies. Do this as and when seeds ripen, from late summer/early autumn onwards. Pick a dry day: any moisture around the seeds might make them rot or go mouldy.

» In late autumn, you can start dividing your perennial plants like echinacea, goldenrod, lady's

james's tip Some people slash back growth now to 'put the garden to bed' for winter, but I don't prune much at colder times of the year because it can cause infections and some dead top growth can actually help protect the healthy tissues underneath. Instead, leave plants to self-seed, and you'll get to see the beauty of white frost on dried seedheads on a winter morning.

mantle, lemon balm and valerian. This will increase your stock and stop clump-tending plants from becoming congested.

» Start taking cuttings from shrubby plants such as bay, blackcurrants, elder, lemon verbena, rosemary and willow from mid-autumn onwards into the winter. (These are called hardwood cuttings.) Plant them in a free-draining seed compost and keep under cover, indoors, or in a conservatory or greenhouse, until next spring.

» Some seeds can now be sown straight out into the garden: angelica, marshmallow, pansy.

» Keep an eye on the weather: you don't want to get caught out by an early frost, or your more delicate plants will suffer. Cover them with horticultural fleece or bring them inside, or into a greenhouse.

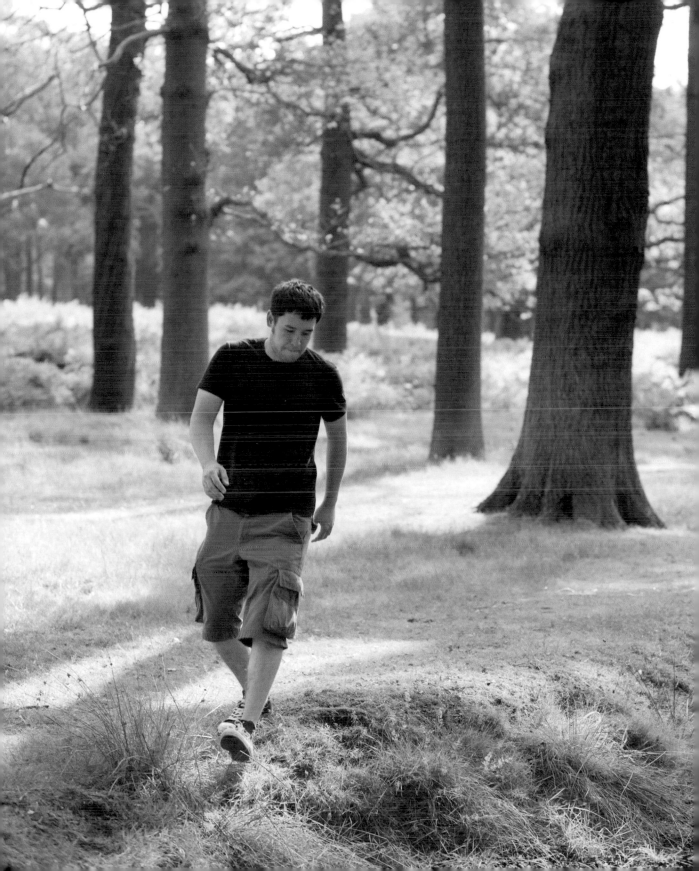

growing fruit trees

It might not be the old, gnarled apple tree you climbed as a child, but you'll be able to grow a fruit tree even in a tiny courtyard garden provided you have some sun at some point during the day.

Many fruit trees are perfect for the smaller garden, including apples, pears, peaches, plums and sweet cherries. These can be pruned and trained to grow flat against a wall in a fan shape or cordon, or as an espalier, a word that means 'shoulder' and describes how the branches are trained to grow out at right angles from the vertical trunk; see opposite.

Fruit trees are traditionally available 'bare-root' in winter, when they are dormant. A good range of trees is also available year-round in containers. Autumn and spring are the best times to plant a fruit tree, but if you can't resist buying a particularly fine-looking specimen in June, don't worry – it'll be fine as long as you keep it well watered at the beginning. (That means every day!) Here's how to plant a fruit tree:

1 Soak the root ball of your fruit tree in a bucket of water for a good few hours prior to planting.

2 Dig a large hole, bigger than the size of the root ball of your plant, to make it easier for the roots to spread out and establish themselves.

3 Add some bulky organic matter, home-made compost, well-rotted manure, mushroom compost or similar into the hole and mix in well.

4 Check the level of the planting hole against the level that the tree is growing in its pot. This is important. The tree must be planted at the same depth as in the pot (or ground if it is a bare-root

james's tip Bag up fallen leaves into bin liners and store over winter for a great soil improver in the spring. Put the leaves in a shredder first; smaller pieces will rot down much more quickly, and you'll have compost in a hurry!

tree). Fruit trees are usually grafted – that is, the top of one tree (grown for its fruit) is joined to the bottom of another tree (grown for its strong roots). If you bury the graft or part of the trunk, you run the risk of damaging or even killing the tree.

5 Once the hole is the right depth, take the tree out of its pot and stand it nice and straight in the hole. (Another pair of hands or eyes is sometimes useful here.) Backfill the hole with soil so the tree is stable but not completely planted yet.

6 Staking is important. Tree stakes and ties are available at all good garden centres and provide support for a young developing tree. Knock a stake into the ground to the side of the root ball (being careful not to drive it through the roots, as this will cause damage).

7 Backfill the planting hole completely and firm well in with the heel of your boot.

8 Tie the tree to its stake. Don't bend the tree – just take a tree tie or a length of old tights and make a figure of eight between the two (this stops rubbing and damage to the trunk). Once the tree has grown a bit, you'll need to check that the ties have not become too tight.

9 Water in well and remember to water the tree every day for a while, especially during summer and dry weather.

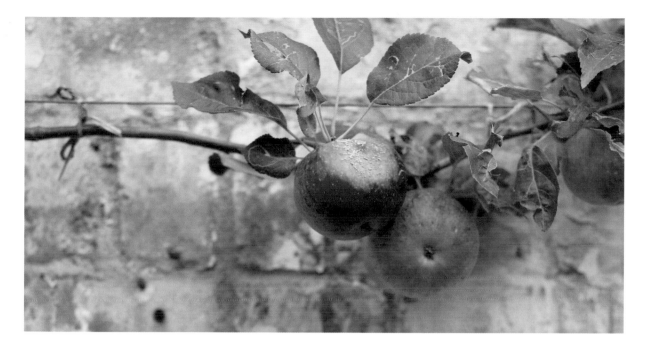

to espalier a fruit tree

You get much more fruit from branches trained laterally or at an angle against a wall – and it also makes better use of limited garden space. You can espalier apple, cherry, pear, peach and plum trees, though you'll need a little patience and some TLC to get the best results. Here's how:

1 Before you start planting, put up some strong horizontal wires on the wall to support the tree's framework, about 30–40cm apart.

2 Plant a bare-root fruit tree as described opposite. You'll need what's called a maiden whip, a single-stemmed tree. Push a cane into the ground behind, and tie the stem to it vertically.

3 Immediately prune the maiden whip just above the first lateral wire, at a point where there is a bud with 2 well-formed buds below it – these will then grow out, one to each side, to produce the first espalier tier, while the top bud forms the vertical stem. Tie the top stem in to the vertical cane as it grows.

4 Tie two canes at an angle of 45º to the stem, one each side, and tie in the first espalier branches as they grow. Once the branches are long enough (which might take a few months), drop the canes down to an angle of 90º along the wire, and tie in firmly. In winter, prune these branches by about one-third to a downward-facing bud.

5 The same winter, form the second tier. Cut the leader stem to just above the second lateral wire, to a place with a bud with two strong buds below it. Follow Step 4 above. Cut back any other lateral branches (apart from the espaliers) to 3–4 leaves.

6 Next winter, form the third tier, following Steps 5 and 4 above.

7 Next summer, you'll be able to harvest a wonderful crop of fruit.

AUTUMN: ROOTS AND RHIZOMES FOR PICKING

The roots can be as powerful medicinally as any other part of the plant. You can use them fresh, though some are more effective when dried, and that way they'll also see you through the year. Roots are best picked when they have been through at least one growing season – and a few like ginseng get more powerful as they mature. Here are a few to look out for.

✱ *The potential health benefits of the plants listed below are based on their traditional use.*

Angelica *Angelica archangelica*, anti-inflammatory, can help relieve flatulence and indigestion, and loosen respiratory catarrh. Harvest year-old roots.

Bistort *Persicaria bistorta*, astringent, anti-diarrhoeal and anti-inflammatory, used to help stop bleeding and reduce catarrh, applied topically to wounds.

Dandelion *Taraxacum officinale*, gentle diuretic, health tonic, anti-inflammatory.

Echinacea *Echinacea angustifolia, E. purpurea* or *E. pallida*, helps stimulate the immune system and lessen the severity and duration of cold and flu symptoms. Harvest 3–4-year-old roots.

Elecampane *Inula helenium*, used to soothe coughs and lung complaints such as bronchitis.

Ginger *Zingiber officinale*, for dyspepsia, nausea and motion sickness, warming. Harvest year-old roots.

AUTUMN: WILD BERRIES FOR PICKING

It's surprising how many berries you can find in the wild in early autumn, for use in health-giving remedies. Here are some of the most common.

✱ *The potential health benefits of the plants listed below are based on their traditional use.*

Blackberries *Rubus fruticosus*, high in vitamin C, mildly astringent and anti-diarrhoeal.

Elderberries *Sambucus nigra*, have antiviral properties and help speed recovery from colds and flu, anti-inflammatory, delicious in jellies. DO NOT EAT RAW.

Goji berries *Lycium barbarum*, can help stimulate the immune system in colds and flu.

Haws *Crataegus monogyna* or *C. laevigata*, tonic for heart health and circulatory diseases.

Juniper berries *Juniperus communis*, diuretic, anti-inflammatory, used to help with urinary tract infections. Pick only black berries – they take 2 years to ripen.

Wild rosehips *Rosa canina*, full of vitamin C, for colds and sore throats, and also used for rheumatism and arthritis.

Ginseng *Panax ginseng*, traditionally used to boost energy and improve physical and mental performance. Harvest roots of 6–7-year-old plants.

Horseradish *Armoracia rusticana*, applied topically for sore muscles and joints.

Liquorice *Glycyrrhiza glabra*, to loosen congestion in coughs and bronchitis, for sore throats, demulcent, soothes stomach inflammation and ulcers. DO NOT TAKE HIGH DOSES OVER A PROLONGED PERIOD.

Marshmallow *Althaea officinale*, contains mucilage to soothe gastrointestinal tract, coughs and sore throats, softening for skin.

Rhubarb *Rheum rhabarbarum, R. rhaponticum* or *R. officinale*, anti-inflammatory and mild laxative, rhizomes used in polish to brighten the colour of wood. DO NOT EAT THE LEAVES, THEY ARE POISONOUS.

Rose root *Rhodiola rosea*, can alleviate low mood and help improve physical and mental performance.

Tormentil *Potentilla erecta*, astringent, traditionally used for sore joints and muscles, internally for diarrhoea and tummy bugs and externally to stem bleeding and heal wounds.

Turmeric *Curcuma longa*, used to soothe arthritic joints and other inflammatory conditions, including those of the skin and digestive system.

Valerian *Valeriana officinalis*, sedative, used to calm anxiety and nervous tension, the dried root is loved by cats.

drying roots

The roots of perennial plants are like rechargeable batteries – once the leafy green bits above the ground have died back, all the plant's active ingredients retreat into its roots.

This makes autumn the best time to pick roots and rhizomes for remedies. With a garden fork, gently prise them up, being careful not to damage them. Give them a good wash to get the soil off, then trim any side shoots or stems. Small roots can be dried whole, but larger roots like horseradish can be sliced in half lengthways first, then cut into regular-sized smaller slices – the idea is to dry each part of the root evenly, so aim to make them all the same thickness and length.

Spread the roots out on baking trays covered with greaseproof paper, and pop them into the oven at the lowest setting (you need a temperature of about 50–60ºC, 120–140º F), leaving the oven door open. Check regularly, turning them occasionally until they have passed the spongy stage and become brittle and dried through but not shrivelled up. (It's hard to be precise about timing, as the moisture content is different depending on the plant and when you harvested it.) Store the dried roots in a dark glass jar, labelled and dated, with an airtight lid until needed. They will keep for up to 1 year.

AUTUMN: SEEDS FOR PICKING

Keep an eye on your seeds – they ripen very fast. You want to pick them for use medicinally just as the seed pods change colour, which is usually at the very tail end of summer and the start of autumn. Here are some to look out for.

✳ *The potential health benefits of the plants listed below are based on their traditional use.*

Angelica *Angelica archangelica*, anti-inflammatory, can help relieve flatulence and indigestion, and loosen respiratory catarrh. Will self-seed in autumn.

Aniseed *Pimpinella anisum*, expectorant used in bronchial conditions, as a digestive soother, kills external parasites such as the scabies mite and lice.

Black mustard *Brassica nigra*, seeds applied topically to encourage circulation and soothe muscle pain.

Caraway *Carum carvi*, to aid digestion.

Celery *Apium graveolens*, anti-inflammatory, to help decrease swelling in gout and arthritis, gently sedative.

Coriander *Coriandrum sativum*, to aid digestion and soothe stomachs.

Dill *Anethum graveolens*, traditionally used for digestion, gas and intestinal spasms; chew seeds to help alleviate bad breath.

Fennel *Foeniculum vulgare*, to ease bloating and stomach upsets, applied topically as an eyewash.

Flax *Linum usitatissimum*, the seeds (known as linseed) are used as a laxative, for coughs and bronchitis, topically for burns, and as a phytoestrogen.

drying seeds

When seed pods start changing colour, give them a quick tap: if the seeds fall onto the ground, they are ready to be harvested and dried.

The easiest way to harvest them is to cut off the seedheads with some stalk still attached. Put a paper bag around the seedheads, and tie it with string around the stalks. Hang the bundle of herbs in a warm, dry, well-ventilated place at a temperature of about 20–32ºC (68–90ºF) – an airing cupboard or warm loft space is ideal. As they dry, the seeds will drop into the bag. Leave them to dry thoroughly for a couple of weeks, then shake the bags hard to catch all the seeds. Pour them out onto a flat tray, removing any seed husks. Store the seeds in paper bags or envelopes, labelled and dated. Most seeds will keep for about 1 year for use in remedies (or sow them next spring), though angelica is viable for only 3 months.

AUTUMN: LEAVES FOR PICKING

There's still quite a lot around to be picked indoors and out, and not just evergreens, either. Avoid yellowing or wilting leaves and go for the brightest green leaves you can find. Here are some to look out for.

james's tip If you have any black mustard plants left over, they're brilliant as a green manure. Dig them into soil at the end of the growing season; they add all sort of goodies and 'fix' nitrogen in the soil, thus making this vital nutrient available to other plants.

⁕ The potential health benefits of the plants listed below are based on their traditional use.

Aloe vera *Aloe barbudensis*, the gel soothes burns and skin problems, speeds healing time of cuts and wounds.

Basil *Ocimum basilicum*, antibacterial, used mostly as an aromatic in aftershaves and colognes.

Bay *Laurus nobilis*, aids digestion, used in aftershaves and colognes for its pungent aroma.

Eucalyptus *Eucalyptus* spp., decongestant for colds and coughs, antiseptic in sore throats and skin treatments, good insect repellent.

Fennel *Foeniculum vulgare*, to ease bloating and stomach upsets, applied topically as an eyewash.

Horsetail *Equisetum arvense*, traditionally used for cystitis and to help improve thin, brittle hair and nails.

Lemon balm *Melissa officinalis*, calming, helps soothe nervous tension and relieve anxiety. Applied topically to treat cold sores.

Mint *Mentha* spp., often used to help with bloating, dyspepsia and irritable bowel syndrome, applied topically as an antiseptic and to soothe itching.

Parsley *Petroselinum crispum*, diuretic, used for digestive problems and anaemia. DO NOT USE IF YOU HAVE KIDNEY PROBLEMS.

Rosemary *Rosmarinus officinalis*, reputed to help memory and concentration and increase alertness. Applied topically for muscle pain.

Sage *Salvia officinalis*, helps loosen mucus in the upper respiratory tract and soothe the throat, used for hot flushes and sweating during menopause.

Thyme *Thymus vulgaris* or wild thyme (*Thymus serpyllum*), antiseptic, especially for the mouth, used to help loosen phlegm, applied topically to ease rheumatic pains, insecticidal.

Watercress *Nasturtium officinale*, vitamin and mineral-rich, general health tonic.

Wild marjoram *Origanum vulgare*, antiseptic used to soothe respiratory and urinary tract infections.

WINTER

Everything has died down now, it's quiet outside, and you can at last put your feet up and get anoraky with the seed catalogues. Perfect, a cup of herbal chai and some armchair gardening ...

This is the time to ...

» Get out the horticultural fleece. It costs only around £1 a metre, and it can be a lifesaver in cold areas of the country for plants prone to frost damage, such as young bay trees, lemon verbena and sage. It basically acts like a thin woolly jumper, trapping a layer of warm air around the plants and providing a barrier to frost. Tie it loosely over small plants when frost is forecast.

» Some plants need more protection than horticultural fleece can provide, and bringing them into an unheated greenhouse, conservatory or indoor windowsill will do the trick. These include aloe vera, citrus trees, ginger, gotu kola, lemongrass and scented-leaved pelargoniums. Olives and the tea bush might be thankful for a break from the harshest conditions too.

» Forget trying to nurse delicate herbs like basil, coriander and tarragon through a British winter:

they'll be weak, prone to attack by pests and disease, and won't thrive for a second year. Treat them as annuals, dig them up and chuck them in the recycling. You can always sow fresh seed next spring.

» Start mulching: choose a cold, sunny day and get stuck in. The garden is now at its emptiest and it'll be easy to spread a generous 5–10cm layer of mulch to keep the weeds down, the moisture in and feed the plants in the coming year. (Use home-made compost, well-rotted manure, mushroom compost, leaf mould – whatever you can get your hands on.) Be careful not to pile mulch around the stems of any plants still visible, as it could burn or damage them.

» Don't forget to water indoor plants occasionally. We can still have warm days in winter and these, together with double glazing and central heating, can catch you out if you are a bit blasé about watering.

» Make fantastic original gifts from your favourite remedies (see page 202).

» This is when I always start geeking out over seed and plant catalogues. It's a good time to think ahead and decide what you're missing in your indoor or outdoor planting space, which nurseries you'd like to use, and which seed companies you're going to try next.

james's tip If the weather catches you out (which happens to even the most seasoned gardener) and you're not fully stocked up with horticultural fleece, an old net curtain or light sheet will do the job just as well.

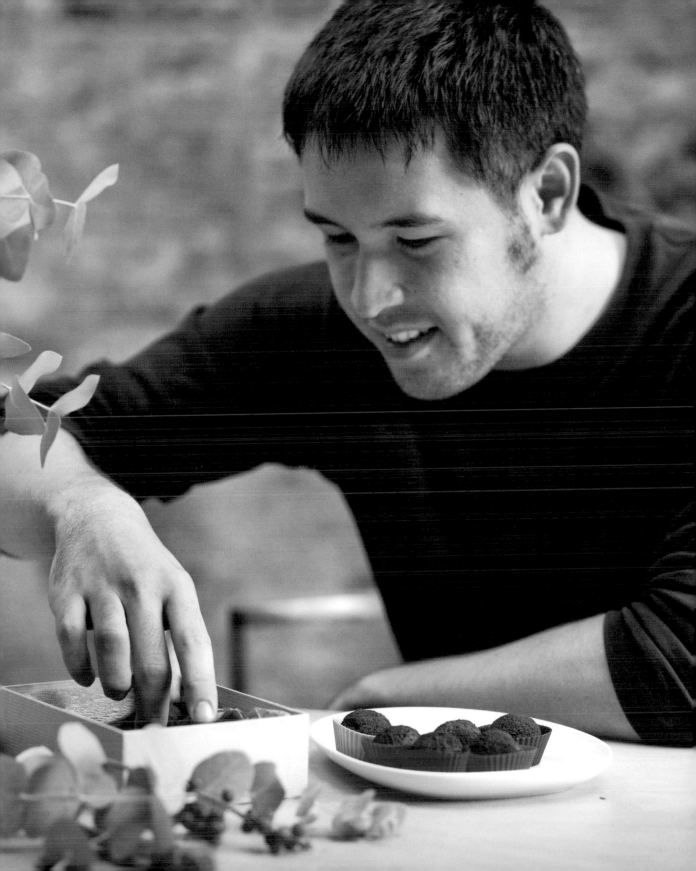

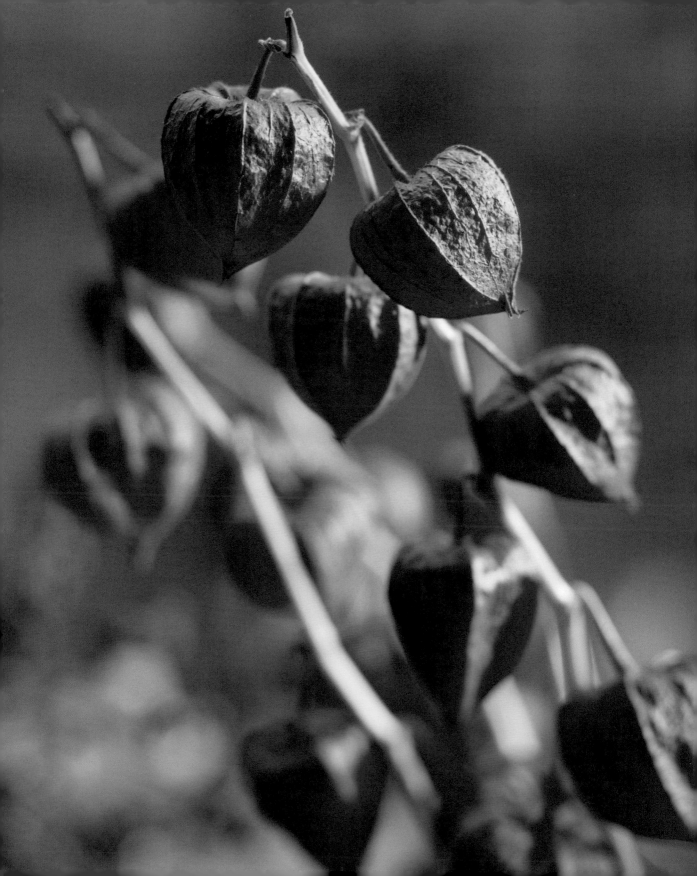

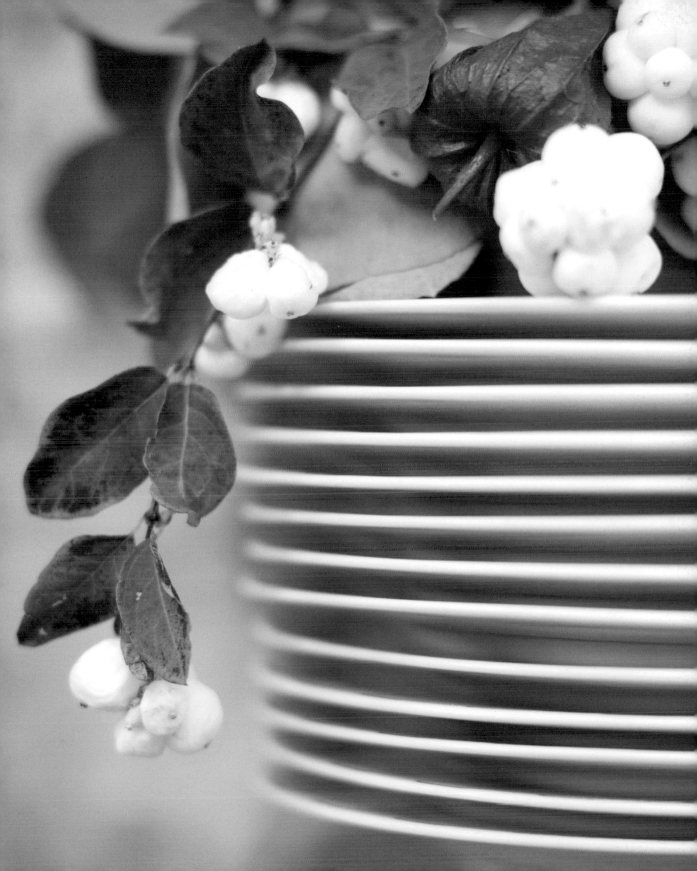

HOW TO GROW A CITRUS TREE

People think citrus are fussy, difficult plants to grow in Britain, but treat them right and you'll be rewarded with a healthy tree that bears a fabulous stock of fruit.

Lemons and limes are generally easier to grow than oranges, but my favourite citrus is the calamondin (*Citrofortunella microcarpa*), which is popular in South-East Asia. It's somewhere between a mandarin orange and a kumquat with unusual, fragrant sweet/sour fruits – weirdly, the skin is sweet and the flesh is sour, so it makes an exotic-tasting combination. Use the juice as you would a lime, or slice the whole fruits and pop them in smoothies, juices or even cooked in syrup – lovely! Despite its origins, it's one of the hardiest of all citrus, so is easier to grow here, and its fruits stay on the tree all year round, which is useful when you want a quick bit of juice or rind for a recipe. Handily, they are also one of the most commonly available of all citrus; check in the houseplants section of your local garden centre. They produce masses of fruit even from a tiny foot-high plant. All citrus are best grown in pots as you can move them around throughout the year – to a sunny, sheltered outdoor spot in summer, and indoors in winter.

1 Choose a large pot, at least 60cm in diameter – citrus are quite slow-growing, so this will be its home for a few years.
2 Plant the tree in a nutrient-rich, loam-based compost. Water in.
3 Keep the pot outdoors in a sunny, sheltered spot from the last frosts in late spring until the first in early autumn, then bring indoors or into a conservatory or unheated greenhouse.

4 Water your citrus regularly through the summer, taking note of the weather: water more in sunny periods and less in wet summers.
5 Give your citrus a liquid feed regularly (up to once a week) during the growing season (spring and summer). This will stop the leaves yellowing, keep the plant growing strongly and make sure the fruits form well.
6 The beautifully scented, creamy-white waxy flowers bloom in late winter, and the fruit ripens up to 12 months later. Because fruits take so long to mature (6–8 months), citrus trees can be in flower and fruit at the same time.
7 Don't be afraid of pruning your lemon, orange or lime tree; it'll thank you for it. Cut back congested growth in late winter or early spring and tidy up stray growth in the summer to keep the shape you like. Remember that if you do a major overhaul you might lose the flowers and fruit for that year. A good feed and water after the pruning will help the tree to recover.
8 To harvest, cut the fruit off at the stalk with a sharp knife, or give it a quick twist.

james's tip In early winter, it's a good idea to raise outdoor containers off the ground to stop them freezing and cracking. You can buy pot feet, but I like to use upturned water or fizzy drink bottle tops instead. Just slide 3 of them, equally spaced, under the pot; you don't see them, so they won't spoil the look of your display, they'll raise the pot a few centimetres above the ground, and you're recycling too.

WINTER: FRESH PLANTS FOR PICKING

The evergreens are still going strong, and many leaves can be picked from indoor and outdoor plants throughout the winter. Here are some to look out for.

* *The potential health benefits of the plants listed below are based on their traditional use.*

Aloe vera *Aloe barbadensis*, the gel soothes burns and skin problems, speeds healing time of cuts and wounds.

Bay *Laurus nobilis*, aids digestion, used in aftershaves and colognes for its pungent aroma.

Eucalyptus *Eucalyptus* spp., decongestant for colds and coughs, antiseptic in sore throats and skin treatments, good insect repellent.

Holly *Ilex paraguariensis* (yerba mate), use as traditional seasonal greenery, can be bought in tea form.

Ivy *Hedera helix*, used in cosmetic treatments to help cellulite. The leaves are used in expectorant cough mixtures. DO NOT EAT THE BERRIES.

Olive *Olea europaea*, oil used as an emollient for skin and in cooking, leaves used for mildly elevated blood pressure and to help control blood sugar levels.

Parsley *Petroselinum crispum*, diuretic, used for digestive problems and anaemia. DO NOT USE IF YOU HAVE KIDNEY PROBLEMS.

Rosemary *Rosmarinus officinalis*, reputed to help memory and concentration and increase alertness. Applied topically for muscle pain.

Sage *Salvia officinalis*, helps loosen mucus in the upper respiratory tract and soothe the throat; used for hot flushes and sweating during menopause.

Thyme *Thymus vulgaris* or wild thyme (*Thymus serpyllum*), antiseptic, especially for the mouth, used to help loosen phlegm, applied topically to ease rheumatic pains, insecticidal.

Witch hazel *Hamamelis virginiana*, used as an anti-inflammatory and to stem bleeding. Leaves and twigs are used to soothe bruises, sprains and skin conditions.

bletting

Just as ripe cheese and wine are tastier than fresh, some fruits are better left to mature on the tree until the first hard frosts arrive.

This is an ancient and once extremely widespread practice called bletting. The intense cold starts a chemical process that breaks down the tannins and increases the sugars in the fruit, giving them a richer, more palatable flavour. Good fruits for bletting include quinces, medlars, sloes and rosehips – after a frost, you'll notice the colour of the rosehips brightens and they soften slightly. This is a great time to get out and pick rosehips for use in syrups rich in vitamin C and medicinal preserves (eat a daily spoonful or spread the jam/jelly on toast). These will help keep everyone healthy over winter.

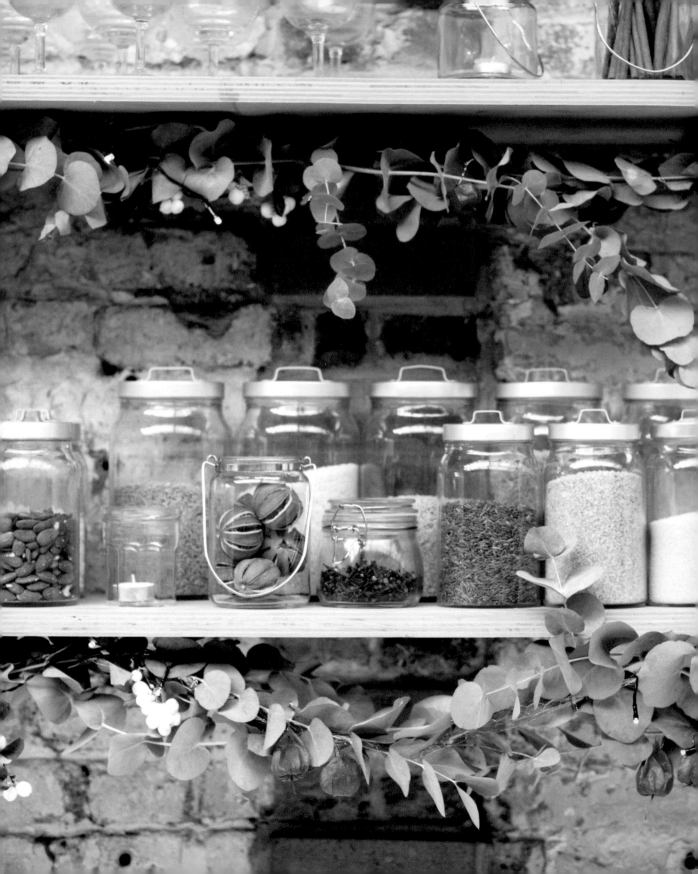

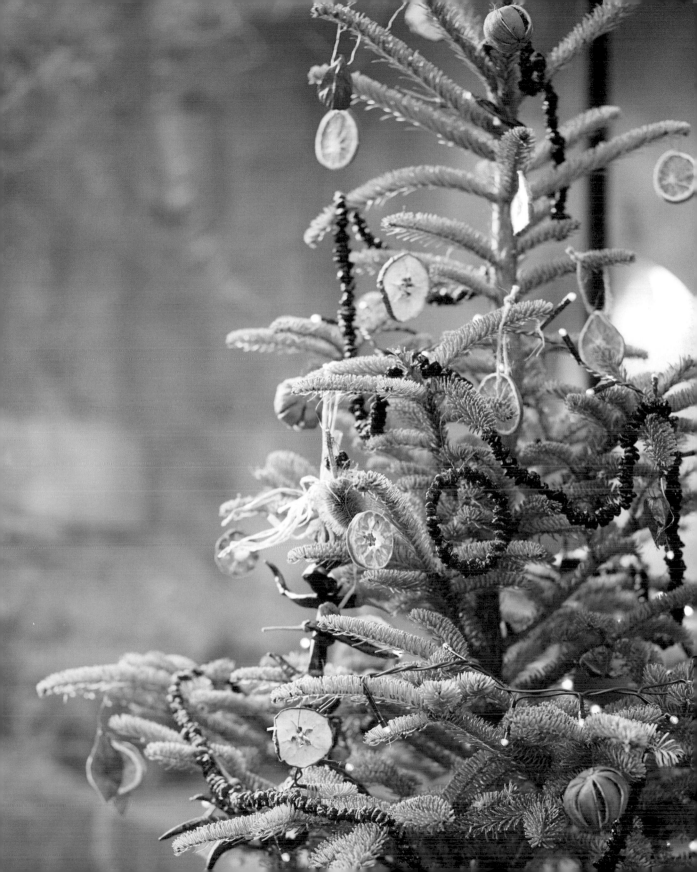

GREAT AS GIFTS

When it comes to present-giving, it's not just the thought but the work-rate that counts, and I don't think you can do better than give someone something you've grown, nurtured and made yourself, and which is also natural, organic and good for them!

Many of these remedies can be dressed up to make the most brilliant gifts – throughout the book, I've put 'gifting flashes' to flag up interesting, creative ways of packaging them into must-have presents for friends, family, work mates and others in your life.

Early winter is the time to get going on the gift-making, so they're ready for the big seasonal present-giving extravaganza in December. Before you get started, you might need a few of the following bits and pieces:

Decorative bottles: I like Kilner jars; they're practical, come in all sizes and always look good. You can recycle old ones or buy new ones in catering supply shops or online, and they'll last for years (you might need to replace the orange plastic seals occasionally). You can find old preserving, pharmacy,

perfume and other decorative bottles and jars in second-hand shops and at car boot sales. (Don't worry if they have crumbly old corks – you can always buy new ones to fit.) Bottles come in a huge range of different shapes and sizes and it depends what you want them for: vinegars and oils look good in tall, clear bottles; tinctures in small, dark glass bottles (black, brown or dark blue). For small dosages, look out for spray, pipette and dropper bottles. The old-fashioned swing tops (as on some beer or lemonade bottles) are good for cordials. Remember to sterilize all recycled bottles before you use them (see page 35).

Jam jars: Recycle old ones – I have a cupboard stashed full of them. You often find quirky hexagonal mustard/sauce jars, which look great as gifts.

Decorative pots and troughs: As well as terracotta, these come in ceramic, stone, wood, enamel, lead, tin, zinc, plastic, wire and fibreglass, shaped as pots, wall containers, urns, planters, cisterns, troughs, coppers, hanging baskets and window boxes. You can make original gifts out of old chimney pots, galvanized buckets, wooden wheelbarrows and porcelain sinks – for example, plant a chamomile 'lawn' in a Victorian ceramic handbasin or make an exotic zinc trough by planting up with succulents. Keep your eyes open for bargains wherever you are – car boot sales, junk and second-hand shops are probably cheapest, but there are wonderful finds at architectural salvage yards and auctions too. Remember that you may need to drill drainage holes in the base of some recycled containers.

Old tin boxes: Great for cough sweets and lozenges. You can find retro boxes in second-hand shops, usually going cheap.

Card: To cut up and make into decorative gift labels. You can buy A1 sheets of good-quality white, cream or coloured card (with plain or textured surfaces) from art shops – way cheaper than buying individual labels. Just cut out a small rectangle whenever you need it, write the label, punch a hole in it, and attach with ribbon.

Ribbon, raffia or string: All look good wound round the neck of bottles and jars, or used to attach labels. Ribbon is pricey, so recycle it whenever you can. (Just give it an iron if it's looking crumpled.)

Cardboard boxes: Don't chuck out any good cardboard or decorative boxes you get given, with lids or without. If they've got brand names on them, revamp them (and the lids) by covering with wrapping paper. Then you can pad them inside with coloured tissue paper and nestle your jars on top. Tie with a big ribbon bow for a luxe look. Alternatively, you can buy colourful cardboard boxes in stationery shops – though these might cost more than your gift.

Cellophane: This gives ordinary gifts the wow factor. Stand your jar or bottle on a big sheet of cellophane, then wrap the cellophane around, gathering it at the top with a ribbon bow. If a gift box doesn't have a lid, stick a cellophane sheet over the top of it to give a professional finish. You can buy bags, as well as clear and coloured cellophane sheets – normally green and red, very seasonal – from kitchen shops. These are great for making up gifts of pot pourri, tea, cough sweets, etc.

some gift ideas:

» A citrus, olive or bay tree in a beautiful pot decorated with a huge bow.

» Make a mini Eden Project by planting up a galvanized zinc trough with green and red succulent plants such as aloe, rose root (*Rhodiola rosea*) and houseleeks. Scatter black slate chippings round for a minimalist look to suit the most modern tastes.

» Infused oils and vinegars (see pages 30–1) – put a fresh sprig of the plant in the bottle to make them even more appealing.

» Health-giving jellies, honeys and jams, with handwritten labels.

» Winter tonics in old-fashioned, wide-necked syrup bottles.

» Cough sweets and lozenges in pretty tins.

» Balms and face and body creams in small blue, black or amber wide-mouthed jars.

» Sweet-smelling body scrubs and bath salts in glass jars.

» A bottle of homemade liqueur presented in a box with a couple of glasses.

» Cordial and 'champagnes' in swing-top bottles.

» Personalized eau de cologne in a beautiful perfume bottle.

» Beautifully stitched moth sachets stuffed with aromatic herbs, for clothes addicts.

» Tins of homemade furniture polish for green home-owners.

» Homemade pot pourri (just mix up your favourite dried aromatic herbs in cellophane bags).

» Ornamental door wreaths made with seasonal greenery, perhaps with some home-grown chillies or eucalyptus berries …

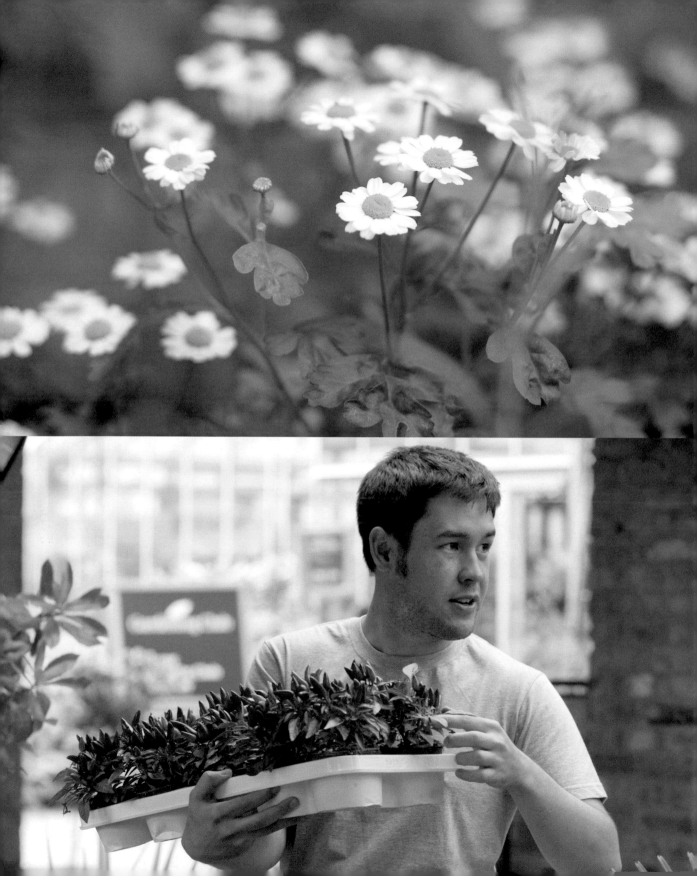

5 THE NON-GARDENER'S GUIDE & RESOURCES

THE NON-GARDENER'S GUIDE

Far too many mates of mine secretly confess that they would love to start gardening but find rigid pruning rules and obscure digging techniques just too daunting a prospect – like a horticultural 'times tables' that you need to memorize before you can even think about getting going.

For the resolute non-gardeners put off by their own lack of skills and horticultural know-how, I would like to say that it's a lot easier than you think – and practice makes perfect! The pay-off is the real thrill you get when your plants eventually grow and flower.

An increasing amount of research suggests that some of the longest-held and widely taught techniques in horticulture, most of which date back to Victorian times, have less scientific basis than first thought. Nowadays, these techniques have been well and truly tried and tested and the nonsense ones disregarded. It seems that Victorian gardeners had a habit of making over-complicated and unnecessary rules to make gardening seem a bit trickier that it really need be, effectively to make themselves appear as horticultural geniuses – a bit like the buzzwords and 'corporate speak' of today's management consultants. In one simple experiment, scientists took a hedge cutter and slashed a straight line through a row of rose bushes instead of painstakingly pruning each branch to the precise length, angle and direction as all 'proper' gardeners have been taught since the 19th century. The bushes with the chainsaw treatment produced far healthier growth and lots more flowers than the conventionally pruned bushes, thereby completely debunking one of the trickiest rules in gardening. Of course, there are also plenty of fantastically useful horticultural tips and tricks, and once mastered these almost guarantee success. As with all rules in life, the trick is to give them a go and see which work for you.

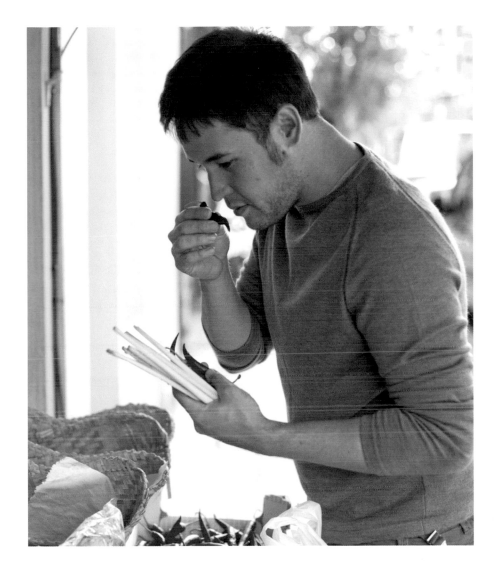

Not only do you not need particularly green fingers, you don't even need a garden. With clever planting choices, the smallest balcony or even a couple of pots on your kitchen windowsill can supply the raw ingredients for a huge array of remedies. But for the truly horticulturally challenged amongst us, there are plenty of alternative ways to get hold of the plants you need without the obligation to grow anything at all. A walk in the countryside, a raid on the gardens of friends and neighbours (a personal favourite of mine), or even a few mouse clicks online can provide you with all you need to create a homemade medicine chest. Especially for the non-gardeners out there, I have set out a guide to help you source and identify good-quality ingredients whatever the time of year – no green fingers necessary.

WILD FORAGING

You don't need to grow the plants for the remedies – many can be found in the most surprising places. If you're looking for a particular plant in the wild, check out the plant distribution maps on the Botanical Society of the British Isles website (www.bsbi.org.uk) before you go to ensure it grows in your area.

in the city

Many hardy plants grow in wasteland and other wild city areas. When you harvest plants for remedies, always pick them away from roads and car pollution. Look out for:

Blackberries, chickweed, dandelion, elder, feverfew, hawthorn, holly, honeysuckle, horseradish, horsetail, ivy, mallow (*Malva sylvestris*, though marshmallow is rarer), nettle, pennyroyal (though it's not prolific), plantain, wild rose (for the hips) and yarrow.

along towpaths

You'll find the following plants along most canal towpaths, even in towns and cities:

Blackberries, dandelion, elder, hawthorn, horsetail, ivy, nettle, plantain and willow.

on chalk downlands

Walking on the downlands and chalky grasslands in southern England, you might spot:

Blackberries, eyebright, hawthorn, vervain, wild marjoram and wild thyme.

hedgerows and meadows

A walk along country hedgerows, lanes and meadows will bring you a bounty of ingredients whatever the time of year. You'll be able to find:

Agrimony, bistort, blackberries, chickweed, dandelion, elder, goji berries (*Lycium barbarum*, in southern England and the Midlands), hawthorn, herb Robert, honeysuckle, horseradish, horsetail, mallow, meadowsweet (in damp areas), mint, mullein, nettle, plantain, St John's wort, valerian, vervain, wild lettuce, wild mustard (including black mustard, in sunny areas), wild rose (for the hips), willow and yarrow.

on heaths and moors

The soil is thin and plants need to be hardy to survive, but on the wild moors, heaths and low mountainous areas in the north of England, Wales and Scotland you can see:

Bilberries (look on the ground – they're low growing), eyebright, goldenrod, rose root (especially in the north), St John's wort, tormentil, wild marjoram and wild thyme.

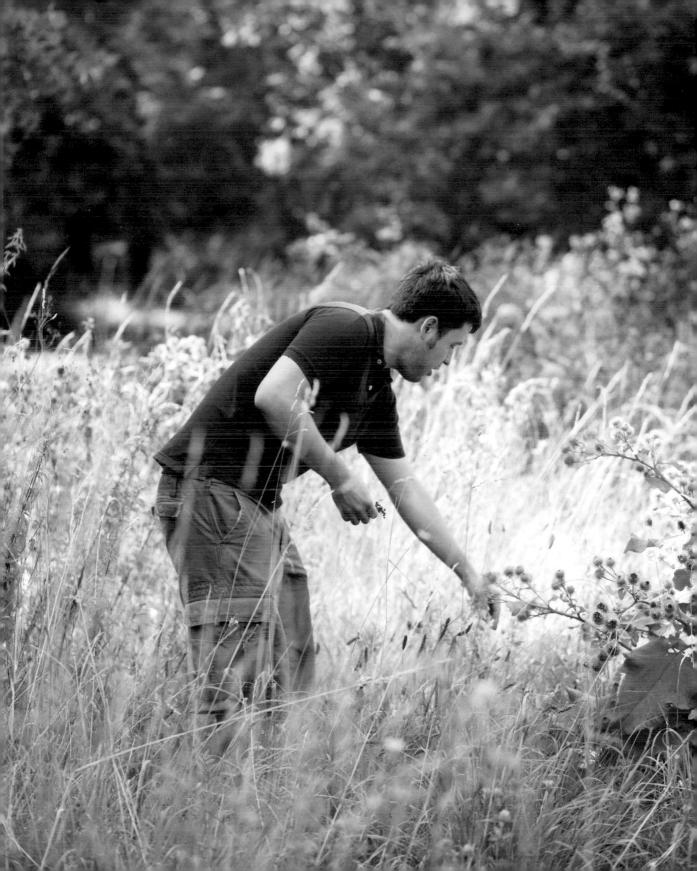

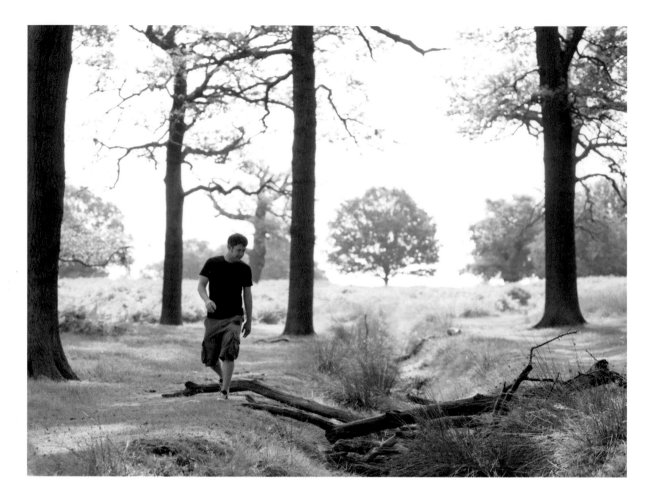

in woodland

On a woodland walk, you'll find a variety of plants and trees – though many, including blackberry, hawthorn and raspberry, tend to grow at woodland margins, where there's more light, rather than deep within. Look out for:

Blackberries, dandelion, elder, hawthorn, holly, honeysuckle, ivy, lime (for the flowers), meadowsweet (near streams and in damp woodland), mint (in damp areas), mistletoe, nettle, pine, raspberries (pick the wild fruits – you can also use the leaves in teas) and willow.

beside the sea

Look out for these plants, which are tolerant of coastal winds, salt spray and sandy dunes:

Elder, fennel, goji berries, juniper, pansy (*Viola tricolor*, in dunes) and wormwood – and, of course, you can find seaweeds such as carrageen and kelp on the beach itself.

FORAGING DOS AND DON'TS

Gathering plants for free on wild land is a great pleasure, but before you get going check you've identified the right plant.

Different species can look very similar – and some lookalike plants can be poisonous. On foraging trips, always take a well-illustrated British wild plant book with you to help with identification. You can pick above-ground growth (foliage, flowers, fruit) of common species for your own use, provided you are not going to sell them on in any form (dried herbs, remedies, jam, jellies, etc.).

You may sometimes need to identify the relevant Local Authority; go to www.direct.gov.uk.

For lists of plants in decline, especially in Wales and Scotland, go to www.plantlife.org.uk. Refer too to the regional rare plant registers and threatened plant database on the website of the Botanical Society of the British Isles: www.bsbi.org.uk.

DO:

» Take a pair of gardening or rubber gloves with you to protect your hands from thorns and nettles. And a bag to put your produce in.
» Pick only the healthiest-looking specimens, avoiding yellowing, diseased or stunted growth.
» Harvest only as much as you are going to use. If you take more than half the green parts of any one plant, you may kill it.
» Get permission from the land's owner (which may be the Local Authority) before you collect any roots from the wild: it is an offence under the Wildlife and Countryside Act 1981 to intentionally uproot any wild plant without permission.
» Ask the Local Authority who looks after the beach for permission before you harvest any seaweed or sand from beaches.

DON'T:

» Pick any wild plant unless you are completely sure you have identified it correctly.
» Pick plants on busy roadsides or from hedgerows alongside cultivated fields where crops are sprayed – you want to avoid exhaust fumes and pesticides when using plants for remedies.
» Harvest from a plant if it is the only one in an area.
» Pick plants that are declining in the wild, such as cornflower, chamomile and juniper.
» Collect excessively from the wild – leave enough to sustain wildlife and ensure plant regeneration.
» Harvest rare or endangered species.
» Pick from Sites of Special Scientific Interest (SSSIs).
» Uproot plants without permission from the landowner.

BUYING PLANTS

Don't worry if you're horticulturally challenged or don't have the time or space to grow anything yourself – you can forage all the plants in this book, some fresh, some dried, and occasionally as oils, from shops ...

asian food stores

When shopping for fresh or dried plants, seeds and other products, have a look in your local Asian or ethnic food shop first – many ingredients are much cheaper there than in health food shops and other specialist suppliers. Look out for:

In the food section: aniseed, black mustard seed, caraway, celery seed, chilli/cayenne pepper, cinnamon, cloves, coriander, cumin, dill seed, fennel seed, garlic, ginger, ginseng, goji berries, lemongrass, linseed, liquorice, nutmeg, tea and turmeric. (You can grow plants from the hardier of these seeds, including goji berries – just plant the seeds from inside the kernel in the dried fruit. Ginger and lemongrass, meanwhile, will root in a glass of water, see page 50.)

In the general section: various oils, including almond, apricot, castor, citronella, coconut, jojoba, olive and safflower, as well as gelatine, glycerine, malt syrup and rosewater.

herbal, health food shops and pharmacies

Here you'll find borax powder, brewer's yeast, friar's balsam (compound benzoin tincture), glycerine, rosewater, vitamin C powder, white petroleum jelly and distilled witch hazel – a key ingredient for the medicine cabinet.

over the counter

The following plants come mostly from tropical and sub-tropical areas and won't grow in Britain's temperate climate.

Most can be sourced from Asian shops and supermarkets, from specialist herbal shops or online. The potential health benefits of the plants listed opposite are based on their traditional use.

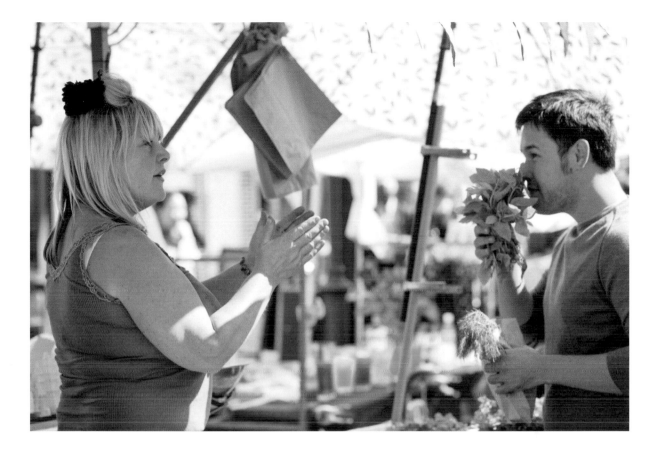

Black pepper *Piper nigrum*, antibacterial and antioxidant, stimulant, digestive, enhances the absorption of medicines and other herbs.

Cardamom *Elettaria cardamomum*, traditionally used to soothe upset stomachs.

Cinnamon *Cinnamomum verum*, analgesic and antioxidant, used to treat nausea, indigestion, colds and flu.

Cloves *Syzygium aromaticum*, used in digestive and respiratory disorders; the oil is antiseptic and analgesic and used for soothing toothache.

Cumin *Cuminum cyminum*, for digestion, colds and fever, antiseptic.

Damiana *Turnera diffusa*, thought to have mood-lifting and stimulating qualities, and reputed to be an aphrodisiac.

Neem oil *Azadirachta indica*, antibacterial and antifungal, used for skin problems, and as an insecticide including for head lice.

Nutmeg *Myristica fragrans*, used for indigestion, nausea and as an anti-inflammatory for stiff joints. TOXIC IN LARGE DOSES.

Quassia tincture *Picrasma excelsa*, insecticide used to treat head lice, bitter stomach tonic in small doses.

Slippery elm powdered bark *Ulmus rubra*, soothing for stomach ulcers, colitis and other digestive disorders.

Tea tree essential oil *Melaleuca alternifolia*, powerful antiseptic and antifungal, used for skin breakouts, cuts and wounds, athlete's foot.

Yerba Mate *Ilex Paraguariensis*, also known as Paraguay holly, mild stimulant and analgesic.

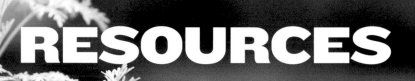

RESOURCES

STOCKISTS

Most of the plant material and other ingredients you'll need are easily available locally, but here are a few online suppliers who stock more specialist items:

Aromantic

www.aromantic.co.uk

Online shop

Bottles and jars, pump/drop dispensers, clay powders, beeswax, vitamin C powder, carrageen seaweed and essential oils. Based in Moray.

G. Baldwin & Co.

020 7703 5550 www.baldwins.co.uk

Shop and online shop

Bottles and jars, pump/drop dispensers, beeswax, emulsifying wax, borax powder, kelp powder, pine, frankincense and myrrh resin, essential oils. Based in London.

Barwinnock Herbs

01465 821338 www.barwinnock.com

Online herb nursery shop

Sells organically grown plants by post. Based in Ayrshire.

Dolphin Sea Vegetable Company

www.irishseaweeds.com

Online shop

Sells a range of seaweeds, including kelp and carrageen.
Based in Belfast.

Emorsgate Seeds

01553 829028 www.wildseed.co.uk

Online shop

Sells a wide range of wildflower seeds. Based near Bath.

Herbs for Healing

01285 851457 www.herbsforhealing.net

Online shop

Herb nursery that sells fresh and dried medicinal plants, pots, jars, bottles, muslin, waxes and specialist oils. Also runs courses on the use of herbs. Based in Gloucestershire.

Jekka's Herb Farm
01454 418878 www.jekkasherbfarm.com
Online shop
Sells a large range of seeds and organic plants
(including specialist plants such as gotu kola).
Based near Bristol.

Landlife Wildflowers
0151 737 1819 www.wildflower.org.uk
Online shop
The environmental charity Landlife sells a wide
range of wildflower seeds. Based in Liverpool.

Laurel Farm Herbs
01728 668223 www.laurelfarmherbs.co.uk
Nursery and online shop
Sells medicinal plants. Based in Suffolk.

Limeburn Nurseries
01275 333399 www.arneherbs.co.uk
Nursery and online shop
Sells medicinal plants. Based in Bristol.

Neal's Yard Remedies
0845 262 3145
www.nealsyardremedies.co.uk
Shops and online
Sells bottles, jars, pump/drop dispensers, beeswax,
emulsifying wax, clay powder, friar's balsam (compound
benzoin tincture), dried herbs, essential oils.

Norfolk Herbs
01362 860812 www.norfolkherbs.co.uk
Online shop
Sells medicinal plants. Based in Norfolk.

Spice World
01984 633685 www.spiceworld.uk.com
Online shop
Sells glass jars, beeswax, vitamin C powder, pine
resin, dried medicinal herbs. Based in Somerset.

Steenbergs Organic
01765 640088 www.steenbergs.co.uk
Online shop
Sells organic dried herbs, unfilled tea bags.
Based in Yorkshire.

Turfshop
01652 678886 www.turfshop.co.uk
Online shop
Sells chamomile turf by the square metre.
Based in Lincolnshire.

PLANT INFORMATION

Botanic Gardens Conservation International
www.bgci.org
A global network of botanic gardens working for plant conservation and undertaking medicinal plant research around the world. Lists botanic gardens in Britain and worldwide.

Botanical Society of the British Isles
www.bsbi.org.uk
Offers flora maps, plant identification guides, archives of botanical publications.

The Herb Society
www.herbsociety.org.uk
Detailed information on the medicinal, culinary and historical uses of herbs.

London Wildlife Trust
www.wildlondon.org.uk
Dedicated to preserving the capital's wildlife and wild spaces.

National Institute of Medical Herbalists
www.nimh.org.uk
The UK's major professional body for medical herbalists.

Natural England
www.naturalengland.org
Protects and conserves English's natural environment and biodiversity.

Plantlife International
www.plantlife.org.uk
Supports wild plant conservation in Britain and internationally.

RHS Plant Finder
www.rhs.org.uk
Database of plant information and gardening advice, with nursery and plant finder tools.

The Wildlife Trusts
www.wildlifetrusts.org
Dedicated to conserving Britain's natural habitat and wildlife environment.

INDEX

Picture Credits

All photographs other than those listed below have been provided by Cristian Barnett.
© Shutterstock 48, 49, 63, 66, 72, 77, 81, 88, 92, 94, 102, 103, 104, 105, 109, 114, 115, 118 (top), 121, 124, 129, 131, 136 (bottom), 137 (bottom), 140, 142, 144 (bottom), 146, 148, 149, 152, 153, 159, 161, 162 (bottom); © Alamy 53, 130 (top), 136 (top), 147, 163; Lucy Hooper and Fino 162 (top)

Author's acknowledgements

Wow, a second book and a follow-up series too. Who would have thought there were so many other like-minded plant geeks out there? I have always thought it was strange though that TV presenters and authors get all the credit, despite the fact that much of the real work is often actually done by a whole army of tireless experts beavering away behind the scenes.

At the front of the charge are Alex Menzies & Lisa Edwards at the BBC for really getting behind the idea 110%. Equally, all the long-suffering team of amazingly talented producers, directors and researchers at Silver River have done a fantastic job. Seriously, some of these guys are so good at what they do that you would think they had been specially created in a lab (you know who you are). Especially big thanks to our ever-effervescent Series Producer, Lucy Hooper, and her team, who have practically bent the laws of physics to ensure that I don't look like too much of a geek on camera!

I am also greatly indebted to the lovely team at HarperCollins for helping put together this brilliant book. I had great fun working on it with them, often involving eating mince pie after mince pie to get the just the right photo to use – my job can be so taxing. Of course none of this would have been possible without the help of our very own pharmaceutical whizz kid, Dr Liz at the University of Reading, whose enthusiasm for concocting all manner of plant based remedies knows no bounds, and an especially huge thank you to Fiona, my excellent agent and unofficial counsellor.

Lastly, a major thanks to all my family and friends for putting up with my geeky plant obsession for all these years, especially my mum who has been the unsuspecting guinea pig for more than one of my lotions and potions.

Publishers' acknowledgements

The publishers would like to thank The Spice Shop, Chiddingfold Forest, Aston Rowant Nature Reserve, Richmond Park, Syon Park Garden Centre and Tilford Cottage Gardens (www.tilfordcottagegarden.co.uk) for their help with photography and Kathryn Lwin Brooks of the Archway Clinic of Herbal Medicine.